Advance Praise for
FIFTY-SEVEN FRIDAYS

"I love this book; this will be one of those rare books that people re-read, think about, and encourage others to read because Myra Sack has somehow been able to put into words the unspeakable, and help us think about the unthinkable by showing us how to bear the unbearable."

–BRUCE D. PERRY, M.D., PH.D, principal of the Neurosequential Network and author, with Oprah Winfrey, of *New York Times* #1 Bestseller *What Happened to You: Conversations on Trauma, Resilience and Healing*

"Required reading for any parent, because it is the story of the greatest love story between a parent and child: loss. The book—beautiful, propulsive, wrenching, and true—reveals the essential truth that there is no love without loss, and that we learn how to love through and within our grief."

–EMILY RAPP BLACK, *New York Times* Best-selling Author of *The Still Point of the Turning World*

"In this beautifully written memoir, we follow the journey of Myra and her husband Matt as they make the excruciating and ultimately life-giving choice to stay fully present with the process of losing their two-year-old daughter Havi to the ravages of Tay-Sachs disease. What struck me most deeply was not only the author's searing authenticity, but Havi's luminous life, her sweet smiles and tender touches, her profound wisdom in the midst of her dying. Death is rarely simple, and the loss of a child will never be okay, yet the love that radiates from these pages has the power to mend the broken world. I will be carrying Havi in my heart forever."

–MIRABAI STARR, author of *God of Love* and *Caravan of No Despair*

"Through the story of the life and death of her young daughter, Havi Lev, Sack shows us with both sorrow and levity that the truest way to honor those we've lost is to hold them close through care and ritual, even after they are gone. This book is both a balm and a manual for anyone who has grieved. I have never read anything like it."

–LAUREN MARKHAM, author of *The Far Away Brothers*

"An act of radical love and profound generosity, *Fifty-Seven Fridays* is required reading. This is the most honest, devastating, and heart-expanding account of what it means to love the one person you're never supposed to lose. Myra Sack does not just shine a light on the inextricable bond between grief and gratitude, anguish and joy, but also provides guidance on how to navigate the impossible. Trust me, Havi Lev Goldstein is about to change your life."

—BECK DOREY-STEIN, *New York Times* **bestselling author of** *From the Corner of the Oval*

"The most incredible memoir... Havi's story will break your heart and mend it bigger than before."

—LISA KEEFAUVER, author of *Grief is a Sneaky Bitch: An Uncensored Guide to Navigating Loss*

"The life Myra Sack depicts in her remarkable memoir is well lived and hard won. In determining to celebrate the life of the beautiful daughter she knows she will soon lose, she calls in love from every quarter—family, friends, community and her readers, too. As heartening as it is sad, as beautiful as it is disturbing this book is an act of grace."

—BEVERLY DONOFRIO, author of *Riding in Cars with Boys*

"Achingly beautiful and wise. *Fifty-Seven Fridays* will transport you to a world where kindness and compassion come alive. Myra's book warmed my soul and I recommend it to all who are curious and seeking nourishment in the form of words."

—ALEXI PAPPAS, Olympian and author of *Bravey*

FIFTY-SEVEN FRIDAYS

LOSING OUR DAUGHTER, FINDING OUR WAY

MYRA SACK

Foreword by
JOANNE CACCIATORE, PhD

Monkfish Book Publishing Company
Rhinebeck, New York

This book is memoir. It reflects the author's present recollections of experiences over time. Some names have been changed *to honor their personhoods and ensure their reputations suffer no harm.*

Hardcover ISBN   978-1-958972-25-0
eBook ISBN 978-1-958972-26-7

Library of Congress Cataloging-in-Publication Data

Names: Sack, Myra, author. | Cacciatore, Joanne, writer of foreword.
Title: Fifty-seven Fridays : losing our daughter, finding our way / Myra
    Sack ; foreword by Joanne Cacciatore, PhD.
Description: Rhinebeck, New York : Monkfish Book Publishing Company, [2024]
Identifiers: LCCN 2023036544 (print) | LCCN 2023036545 (ebook) | ISBN
    9781958972250 (hardcover) | ISBN 9781958972267 (ebook)
Subjects: LCSH: Goldstein, Havi, 2018-2021. | Sack, Myra. | Tay-Sachs
    disease--Patients--Massachusetts--Biography. | Parents of terminally ill
    children--Massachusetts--Biography. | Parent and child. | Terminally ill
    children--Family relationships.
Classification: LCC RJ399.T36 G65 2024 (print) | LCC RJ399.T36 (ebook) |
    DDC 618.928588450092--dc23/eng/20230901
LC record available at https://lccn.loc.gov/2023036544
LC ebook record available at https://lccn.loc.gov/2023036545

Book and cover design by Colin Rolfe
Cover illustration by Abby Hanna & Colin Rolfe

Monkfish Book Publishing Company
22 East Market Street, Suite 304
Rhinebeck, New York 12572
(845) 876-4861
monkfishpublishing.com

Printed in Canada

For Havi, Kaia, and Ezra.
And their Dad.

CONTENTS

PART IV

FOREWORD

Every nook and cranny of grief is hallowed ground. Yet, this hallowed space is sometimes overlaid with the complexities of modernity, social pressure to "move on" from grief, demands on our time, the medicalization (diagnosing grief as a mental disorder) of grief, and past wounds that quietly follow the unawakened heart. These factors, and more, make it difficult to know how to grieve without questioning, even doubting, the wisdom of a broken heart. To grieve honestly and openly—without succumbing to the pressures of society to relegate grief to the margins—is an act of great courage.

Havi's life—and death—are revered with such courage, and much more, in Myra Sack's memoir, *Fifty-Seven Fridays*.

There exist few guides of substantial depth and breadth that help grievers navigate the ebb and flow of emotions when a child dies. *Fifty-Seven Fridays* is a rare gift of intimacy with grief, bringing the reader to a deeper understanding of what it means to fully inhabit—and be unwillingly transformed—by grief. Rather than an emotionally photoshopped exploration of what it means to lose a child, this book is for seekers, for those who wish to understand the nuances and complexities of grief *from the inside*:

> I'm not doing well with any of it. I guess that's expected. The thing is, we are okay right now, in these present moments, because we have you with us physically. You are here: We scoop you up every morning; we place you in between us and snuggle you up in our bed; we hold you for all your meals; we dance with you; we kiss you a thousand times every day; and we tuck you in and sing you to sleep every night. And even as you lose everything, having your warm body curled up in our arms makes it possible to get through a day. And the thing is, in what I call "the long long," I know, or at least I hope, we'll be okay even when we don't have you physically.

> I see amazing people...whose lives are rich, beautiful, filled
> with love, and full of pain, and they all seem okay. But Hav
> girl, what lies in between these two, in between the present
> and the long long, is dark, painful, and uncertain, and that
> scares me. Because the truth is, losing you will never be okay.

Yes, losing a child is complex, excruciatingly so.

While many realize this idiom of truth, at least in the mind, the serious practice of fully inhabited grief is often more elusive in our grief avoidant culture. Myra models this full inhabitation of grief for the reader in such a profound way that fear is dispelled. She invites our hearts to soften and open to the idea that *"forever is right now."* She bids readers into a space of being with grief, layer after layer, from the abstract to the practical, synthesizing sorrow and love, ancient and au courant wisdom. Myra does not offer up short cuts. She doesn't candy coat with superficialities or bypasses. Rather she invites readers along with her and Matt as they commit to the essential and important work of grieving for Havi and learning to parent her, not in the way they want, but in the only way they now can. This is integration, and this is also the tragedy of such loss.

> I feel the one-year anniversary of your death looming and
> I'm afraid of it. My mind is caught in a fog of disbelief. I'm
> afraid of being leveled by the intensity of revisited emotions,
> of the summoning of visceral memories of your last weeks,
> days, and breaths with us. But I'm also afraid that I won't
> feel enough—that I won't feel the pain deep enough or full
> enough. And I don't want to be numb, even if it's just a little
> bit around the edges.

Perhaps one of the greatest challenges facing our inner life as humans today is what the renowned analyst Robert Stolorow calls the "war on emotions." In our happiness-cult society that decries painful emotions like grief, sadness, anger, guilt, and despair, labeling them explicitly or implicitly as pathological, how does a human not *dis*integrate? How does a person reconcile aspects of emotion that the dominant culture overtly rejects? How do we stay with the pain of others, including our intimate partner, if we cannot stay with our own pain?

In order to fully integrate our emotions, and thus be available for the spaces between self and other, we must be aware of them. Awareness of emotions comes from noticing patterns, habits, and both external and internal sensations that are linked to feelings. Myra takes on these issues both explicitly and implicitly through her honest portrayal of grief, gently calling on readers to, not only become acquainted with grief but also, befriend grief, accepting it as part of love, in lieu of trying to control, dispel, or manage grief. The brilliance of her writing is in its nuanced invitation toward emotional intimacy with grief and the burgeoning sense of purpose, that must unfold in its own time, in the aftermath of tragedy.

> If I am here on earth without Havi, I thought, then I owe it
> to both of us to try to have an effect on the world beyond my
> own family, my own little community.

Ultimately, *Fifty-Seven Fridays* is a book about unconditional grief and unconditional love. It's about parenting a child who is dying and then who dies. It's about maintaining connections beyond this world. Fully inhabited grief is one of the most important things we can practice to welcome more authentic and sorrowfully beautiful lives. My life is better for having read this book. And my life is better for knowing Havi. Yours will be too.

JOANNE CACCIATORE, PHD

PROLOGUE

"I think he wants to be my friend, probably wants to go on some runs together," I insist, countering the more suggestive lilt of my mom's query about our "date" later that night. Matt is the older brother of my college soccer teammate, Maggie. We reconnect a few days earlier when Maggie and I run a marathon together. I have just moved from Philadelphia to San Francisco, and I figure Matt is taking me under his wing. I am twenty-three years old and trying to get my footing in a new city.

Long pause.

"Okay, Sweetie," Mom says finally. "Have fun tonight."

We are to start the night at a West Portal bar watching the St. Louis Cardinals play the Texas Rangers in the 2011 World Series. I grab a light jacket, catch the No. 43 bus, and walk a few blocks to the bar. Outside, I fumble in my bag for a piece of gum and my deodorant, which I apply, quickly, on the sidewalk, before heading inside. It is October in San Francisco and I have worked up a sweat between the bus ride and brisk walk.

Matt is poised at a high-top table with a beer. He is wearing jeans and a sharply pressed white button-down that enhances his dark brown hair and eyes and his olive skin tone. He is so cute. And so well dressed. (I wear washed-out jeans, Danskos, and a pale green, off-brand sweater that I've had since middle school.) He stands up, we hug, and I join him at the table.

We duck out of the bar before the game is over. Matt bought tickets to see *Moneyball* at a cool little independent movie theater down the street. San Francisco's famous fog starts to roll in and the streetlights have turned on. The theater is warm and cozy and nearly empty when we arrive. We sit in the middle of a long, empty row. We don't hold hands. Our arms touch, though. And we intermittently exchange glances during particularly poignant parts of the movie. *Moneyball* is about the beauty and heartache that come with team sports. We are both hooked.

"So, what leadership lessons did you take from Billy Beane?" Matt asks before he even starts the car to head home. Billy Beane is the real-life character played by Brad Pitt in the movie. Oh boy. I switch on. This answer feels important. Matt is smart, a Stanford-trained doctor and a clear thinker. I begin sifting my thoughts but can't organize them to my liking. So, I pivot: "Oh, are we in seminar now?!" I joke. "That was a quick transition back to the classroom." He belly laughs. Thank goodness he doesn't take himself too seriously.

We pull up to my apartment on Hayes and Central and Matt gets out of the car to give me a hug. "This was a lot of fun," he says. "Let's do it again sometime?"

"Yeah, whenever works. Drive safe."

I walk inside, sit down at the kitchen table, open a carton of coffee ice cream, and wonder what has just happened. Maggie's older brother. We have already known each other for five years, but things are different now. I like him. I like the way he thinks and the way he communicates. And I like the way I feel with him. But I'm sure this is nothing. He's older, and too handsome, with too many degrees.

* * *

A lot happens between my first date with Matt on that October night in 2011 and September 4, 2016. But in sum, a Philly girl and a Cali boy fall in love, move to Boston, and start a life together.

We choose a family camp in Vermont for our wedding venue and hold our closest people hostage for a three-day weekend of celebrating. We exchange our vows under a chuppah encircled by everyone who matters to us.

September 4, 2018

Two years later, to the day, I stand at the end of a hospital bed with my hands wide on the frame. The contractions are massive now. With each wave my body sinks downward into a deep squat and my screams become a roar. I lie back on the bed for the final push. I see Matt's eyes get teary as the little furry head starts to crest out of me.

And then, at 12:28 p.m.—I can still see the clock on the wall to my left—our baby daughter arrives. Matt catches her. The nurse places her on my chest. Matt stands next to me. We both cry. We can't take our eyes off her.

Our baby is beautiful. Perfect, actually, according to our midwife and nurse. Clear skin, big eyes, strong neck. We name her Havi. The name Havi feels playful and light to us. Havi comes from the Hebrew names Hava and Chai, both of which mean life.

Our world is completely different now. Bigger, better, and also sacred. Everything that matters is in this labor and delivery room. I no longer exist just for me, but for the sake of another human being whose life I will sustain. I want to reach out and hug and kiss every single mom who has ever walked this earth. Motherhood seems like the most overwhelmingly beautiful and daunting task. I have never felt at once so powerful or important, or so vulnerable and scared, all at the same time.

PART
I

"In this short Life that only lasts an hour
How much – how little – is within our power."
EMILY DICKINSON

CHAPTER I

Sleep

April 4, 2018. Havi is seven months old.

"Sleep-train her! You have to, if you want to survive." My new-mom friends, Katie and Juliet, and I are walking our second lap around Jamaica Pond, passing the boathouses, hopscotching around young children on scooters and bikes.

"It took three nights. Now Kyle sleeps through the night," Katie boasts.

"It took a week for us, but Jack aced Ferber," Juliet says, peering around me at Katie in a transparent bid for Katie's approval.

"I've tried it all," I say grimly. "Havi hates being left alone."

"Trust us!" the two moms declare in unison. "What baby wouldn't cry if they know crying gets them nursed and cuddled? The longer you wait, the harder it gets. Stop taking her out of the crib at night!"

* * *

"Do you hear her?" Matt mumbles, rolling toward me in our bed.

"It's my night. I'll go." I glance at the time on my phone. It's 1:15 a.m.

I kick my legs out from under the covers and plant my feet on the floor, jealous that Matt can roll over and go back to sleep. I'm proud of being the only person who can sustain Havi's life. And I'm also exhausted. It's been seven months of little-to-no sleep every night.

I lean over to scoop Havi out of the crib. "I'm here, sweetie." As I cup the bottom of her swaddle, my hands get drenched in pee-poop.

John Legend's "Pampers Lullaby" has become a staple in our middle-of-the-night routine. *Somebody's got a stinky booty, and her name is Havi, and she made a doody.*

She'll grow out of this phase, I tell myself. They don't poop through the night forever. "Okay, beauty girl. Clean diaper, dry onesie, new swaddle. Let's get you fed and back to sleep."

Cradling Havi, I sink into the white rocking chair in the corner. I test my right breast for fullness, then the left, rest Havi's head in the crook of my right arm and drape her body across my legs. The gentle rainlike hum from Havi's sound machine, her lavender-scented calendula lotion, and the perfectly dark room coax me into a pseudo sleep. I fight it, though, knowing it's not safe to sleep with a baby in a chair. Havi's safety has become my preoccupation.

Havi's breathing changes. I ease my nipple from her mouth, rest her body upright against mine, burp her, and lay her back down in the crib. I slowly step away, careful to avoid the creaky spot in the floorboards that always startles Havi awake. I step on a newly creaky floorboard. Havi stirs and cries. Now her left leg is stuck through the crib's bars.

What child wouldn't cry if they knew—*oh, fuck it*. I scoop her up and we settle back down together in the rocking chair for the next few hours, until I try the crib transfer again.

Eventually, I crawl back into bed. "How'd she do?" Matt asks sleepily, clearly oblivious to how long I've been gone. I tap my phone screen: 4:45 a.m.

"She did great," I say. In exactly forty-five minutes, Matt has to get up and go to work. No point worrying him. I'm worried enough for two.

CHAPTER 2

Developmental Delay

September 1, 2019. Havi is three days from her first birthday.

Matt stands over the stove, sautéing onions. Since autumn's chill fell on Boston, he's taken to cooking big pots of delicious pasta several times a week. I sit on the kitchen floor, watching Havi try to crawl toward her reflection in the oven door.

"It looks like she's moving through quicksand," I say. "Crawling shouldn't be this hard for her. Babe, I really think something's wrong."

"She's making steady progress. A little bit every day. She'll get there," Matt reassures me. As I watch, Havi's head drops. Her arms collapse, landing her chest flat on the floor.

I scoop her up. Matt puts down the wooden spoon and spins the two of us around to Fleetwood Mac's "Landslide" issuing from the kitchen speakers. I want to take comfort from Matt's embrace and Havi's soft cheek against mine. But my worries are playing on repeat.

Two months ago, at Logan Airport waiting to board a flight to California to visit Matt's parents, Grandma and Grandpa, Havi sat on the floor at my feet. Nearby, a baby who looked to be about Havi's age was crawling across the industrial gray carpet so nimbly and so quickly, it seemed almost freakish. I couldn't stop staring. His mom kept jumping up to retrieve him.

"How old is yours?" she asked me.

"Ten months," I answered, struggling to keep the fear out of my voice. It felt rude not to return the question and I didn't want to hear the answer. "What about your son?"

"Eight and a half months. An early-crawler!" A flicker of pity crossed her face. "Don't worry, she'll get there. And then you'll miss the days when you could eat a sandwich in peace." I faked a laugh.

"I'm sure you're right," I lied.

Today I remind myself to stay positive. Havi can feed herself; her posture is perfect. When she sits on her own, she looks her age. She smiles at us and laughs deeply. Sometimes she sleeps several hours in a row. Just be patient.

September 4, 2019. Havi is one year old.

It's Havi's first birthday and Matt and my third wedding anniversary, and we're "celebrating" at her pediatrician's office. As always, when we bring her in for a checkup, Matt and I are bursting with pride and excitement. Havi is obviously the most beautiful child on earth, with her sparkling hazel green eyes and her calm, wise demeanor. The office staffers ooh and aah, confirming our diagnosis.

At Havi's nine-month exam, Dr. Richmond examined her heart, lungs, and ears; tested her reflexes; measured her head; checked every inch of her skin; and pronounced Havi "perfect." The same doctor had made the same pronouncement after each exam, starting on Havi's third day of life. I wanted to believe that Havi was perfect, too. But deep down, where my greatest fears lived, I'd started to worry about her development. At twelve months, Havi isn't pulling herself up the way one-year-olds do. She doesn't babble much. She has crawled a couple of times, for three or four strides to retrieve a piece of challah, but she has seemed to be struggling.

I unzip and rezip my jacket nervously as Dr. Richmond examines Havi's little naked body. Finally, she says, "I'm a bit surprised that Havi isn't making sounds or crawling—the normal milestones for her age."

My heart freezes. I grab Matt's hand. His hand is cold.

"We call this developmental delay," Dr. Richmond adds. "It's very common, and Massachusetts has lots of resources to give these types of kids some extra help. I'll also make a few referrals to neurology and orthopedics." Dr. Richmond glances at Matt, then at me. "It's standard protocol," she says. "Nothing to worry about."

These types of kids. The phrase stuns me.

"Here are the numbers to call to start the early intervention." The doctor hands a brochure to Matt. Do I look too freaked out to be a competent parent? I wonder.

Matt and I pack up Havi's bag, get her dressed, and speed-walk to the car. I strap Havi into her seat and strap myself in next to her. Matt takes the wheel. He hands me the brochure.

I lean forward to talk to Matt. "I *knew* she was behind. I don't get it, though. Do you? And why is all of this happening now? Richmond didn't see anything like this." I'm starting to spin. "Are you worried, M?"

"I don't think so," Matt reassures me. "She said Havi's condition is common. And we'll have access to plenty of resources. We'll get a team in place. Can you make that call now, babe?"

"I'm on it," I say, dialing.

By the time we pull into our driveway, we've contacted each of Dr. Richmond's referrals. Matt and I are locked in, fully focused on doing whatever Havi needs.

Over the next few days, our to-do list becomes our fulltime job. Still, each day the list grows longer.

* * *

Eight days after Havi's first birthday, Matt, Havi, and I sit in our family room surrounded by four pediatric developmental specialists, all women, who have come to do an evaluation of Havi.

Since they walked through our front door, greeting the three of us with big smiles and reassuring glances, I've felt like maybe we're going to be okay. Katie leads the meeting. She explains that Havi will be evaluated in five domains: adaptive, personal-social, communication, motor, and cognition.

The four women unpack their bags. A bell, Cheerios, a blanket, a book, and Flexi cups make their way onto Havi's playmat.

As the testing proceeds, I wonder how Havi is scoring. My maternal instincts are on full display, though. I can't seem to keep myself from chiming in on my daughter's behalf. "She can usually pick up a Cheerio from the floor." "Yesterday she lifted her bottle without any help from me."

"We have to see it for ourselves in order to count it," Katie tells me gently.

After three hours under evaluation, Havi starts to fuss.

"We've got what we need," Katie says. "We'll get out of your hair."

Nervously, I ask if she can share the results with us now. Katie promises to email us a full report tomorrow. "But I'm fairly sure that Havi will be eligible for early intervention. In Massachusetts, there's no cost to your family for these services. Havi will likely see a combination of providers—a physical therapist, speech-language pathologist, occupational therapist. She's eligible till she's three years old."

When the door closes behind the developmental specialists, Matt, Havi, and I huddle together in silence. An hour later, I cry in the shower. I don't want Havi to be eligible for an early intervention team. I want her to be eligible for a regular team.

The report arrives in our inbox the next day.

CRITERION CHILD ENRICHMENT

Dear Myra and Matt,
Below is a summary of our findings. Please reach out to us with any questions. We look forward to working with your family.

███████████

Program Director

FINDINGS

Adaptive: Unable to hold bottle up to her mouth by herself.

Personal-social: Able to distinguish between familiar and unfamiliar people. Slow to warm to us, but eventually did. Enjoys being read to and enjoys frolic play.

Communication: Responded to bell from the left to right. Attends to person talking for at least ten seconds. Produces some grunts and sounds.

Motor: Not yet able to crawl. When stands, locks her knees. Raked a Cheerio from the floor.

Cognition: Able to follow a visual stimulus. Aware of new situations. Attended to evaluator when making gestures, but not yet able to imitate.

Summary: Havi is eligible for early intervention in adaptive, communication, and motor. Family has a referral to neurology to rule out anything neurologic.

Havi's personal-social and cognition domains are on track, Matt and I comfort each other. The rest will come. But I can't sleep that night. I toss and turn and agonize. How did we get here? Did I run too much while I was pregnant? Did I miss a few days of prenatal vitamins? Eat too little iron? Did I go back to work too soon? Is our house not set up properly for a baby to learn to crawl or pull herself up?

Tia, our nanny, is wonderful in every way. But maybe Havi needs to hear more English. Or a playgroup so she can spend time with other one-year-olds? Maybe she isn't getting the kind of role-modeling she needs to learn how to babble and crawl.

I need to be near Havi. I creep out of bed and into her room, snuggle up in the rocking chair, watching her sleep. She is still. Peaceful. What could be wrong with this perfect child?

I leave Havi's room and crawl into bed with Matt. His eyes are wide open, staring up at the ceiling. I move to be closer to him.

"I'm scared," Matt says. "What is going on with her? I hated seeing her struggle like that."

"Me too," I agree. "I don't know, lovey. But we'll figure this out. We've got all the right pieces in place now." I say what I think Matt would say, if Matt wasn't too scared to say it himself.

Matt always figures out how to fix everything. Trained as a physician-scientist, he's dedicated his life to healing really sick people. He designs clinical trials for cancer patients. He believes in the power of medicine to save lives. If anyone can navigate this, it's Matt. But I hate that he has to be both Havi's doctor and her dad. I wish he could just be Havi's dad.

I hear Matt's breathing change. He lets out a soft snore. At least *he's* asleep. I roll over, touching my butt to his so we can sleep "butt to butt," as he and I joke. But it takes me a long time to drift off.

* * *

A few days later, Matt, Havi, Tia, and I head to Boston Children's Hospital for Havi's neurology appointment.

In a tiny exam room on the eleventh floor, while we wait for the doctor, Havi sits on the exam table and the three of us take turns playing with her. Tia sings songs and blows bubbles that make Havi giggle. The blissful sounds bubble up from her belly, echoing down the hall. When Dr. Fairweather walks into the room, he's already charmed. He tells us Havi's laughter reassures him. He's seen thousands of one-year-olds with severe and limiting diagnoses. Havi, he says, is clearly not one of them.

We leave Boston Children's that day feeling that a huge weight has been lifted from us. To celebrate, we go to dinner on the patio of a restaurant near home. Each of us orders a glass of wine. "To Havi," we toast. She smiles up at us. Matt and I reminisce about our early dinner dates, when the two of us would split a full bottle of wine. Those carefree days feel like another lifetime now. We pay the check and walk to the car, Matt holding Havi high up on his chest so their eyes are in constant contact. We pull out of the parking lot reminding each other that Dr. Fairweather has given us a reprieve from worrying. After we get Havi to sleep, Matt and I fall into bed feeling like we can breathe again. In the dark, Matt pulls me toward him and we make beautiful love.

* * *

At my younger sister, Leah's wedding, Matt carries Havi down the aisle. I hold his left hand with my right hand, throwing Havi's flower petals for her with my left. Matt and I take our seats.

"I thought she'd run down the aisle ahead of us," I whisper to Matt. He squeezes my leg, "I know, me too. She will, baby. She's making progress every day."

I want to believe him. But I don't.

CHAPTER 3

Pregnant and Afraid

October 1, 2019. Havi is thirteen months old.

"Emmy, Emmy!" I jab at Matt's sleeping body, calling him by my pet name. "It's positive! Look! Can you see the double lines?"

In one move, Matt wakes up, leaps out of bed, and grabs the pregnancy test stick.

"Wow!" he bursts out. "Wow. Wow!"

Matt and I cry. We cuddle. We talk. We cry some more. Matt's breathing turns to snoring. I stare into the blackness. I'm excited to be pregnant again. And I'm terrified about Havi. The path ahead looks turbulent and uncertain.

I struggle to summon hope. Maybe sibling love will be a salve for Havi's younger sibling. For sure he or she will know empathy. Taking care of an older sibling with developmental delay will do that. I start to make a list of families I know whose situations are like ours. Maybe I'll call them. Maybe that will help.

* * *

I race home from work to take Havi to the park. I've done so little of that kind of thing over these past few stressful months, I've been starting to hate myself for it. I walk through the door, send Tia home early, and bundle Havi up. We walk the half-mile to the nearby Tot-Lot, a family-junkyard-turned-kids'-paradise, stocked by neighborhood parents with their kids' cast-off plastic toys, scooters, and play-kitchens. The park is teeming with red-nosed toddlers.

As I lift Havi out of her stroller, my chest tightens. I put her on a small tricycle near two other kids who are cruising around. Havi's feet easily touch the ground, but the bike doesn't move. Her upper body wobbles.

She's about to fall off the bike. Before that happens, I scoop her up and perch her on my hip. "Oh, you want to start with the swings?" I say loudly. I'm lying because I'm embarrassed. I plant a fake smile on my face and walk Havi to the swings. My eyes well with tears. My legs are heavy. I push Havi back and forth, but I'm somewhere else.

At home I find Matt in the kitchen, roasting a chicken.

"I hate the park. She couldn't fucking do anything there."

"Nothing? What about the swing?"

"What's this?" I say, changing the subject, picking up a journal that's open on the kitchen table, its pages covered with Matt's handwriting.

"I think we should start writing to Havi. Document her first year of life."

"Can I read what you wrote?"

Matt nods.

November 11, 2019

Hi, Love of Our Lives,

Do you know how much we love you?

Someday I'm sure your mom and you and I will talk about this year. I picture us laughing about it someday over a glass of wine. In your most adorable fashion, you've decided to take your time doing stuff. We've got a whole army of people helping out with exercises and skills.

You've made some really good progress the last few weeks and I'm so proud of you. You eat with two hands now, more your right than your left, but your left is coming along. And your core is getting stronger—you can balance on the ball or on my knee and when we sit you close to the table you've started to pull yourself up a bit which is really great. You're starting to explore more with your sparkling eyes. It melts my heart when you look at me and smile.

I'm grateful that Matt bought the journal, and I'm grateful for Matt. Our partnership is making this upsetting time doable for me. The journal is a perfect example of the wonderful husband I have. I'd been feeling guilty for not recording more of Havi's life. As usual, Matt found a way to start something beautiful, even in the midst of uncertainty.

November, 2019. Havi is fourteen months old.

Havi's training program is underway. Each day she has a physical or occupational therapy session in our living room, courtesy of home care from Massachusetts State. We bring her to an early intervention playgroup three times a week, and to three additional weekly sessions of physical and occupational therapy at the Boston Ability Center, a private clinic. Matt and I have been succeeding our entire lives. We're both confident that we'll succeed at this, too.

Havi is giving it her all. As painful and frustrating as it must be for her, she struggles through every exercise and never seems to get upset. She does baby crunches on an exercise ball to strengthen her core; pull-ups from a seated position to standing; lies on her belly in front of a plastic doll house to motivate her to raise her head and strengthen her neck muscles. We do exactly as the physical therapist recommends. We start dressing her in reinforced support shorts for babies with low muscle tone. We have her fitted for AFOs (ankle foot orthotics), plastic braces that slide over her feet and up her calf to help her stand.

None of this seems to help.

And it's starting to feel like we're torturing our baby.

There are passing moments when she seems to be making progress—moments that give us hope. But then at a November dinner, when Havi is fourteen months old, I see her slouching in her high-chair. "She needs a pillow behind her back, Emmy. She's tilting in her chair." Matt grabs a throw pillow from a kitchen chair and uses it to prop Havi up.

"Here, sweet girl. Is this better?" Matt turns to me. "I think we need a second opinion. This isn't right. She's going in the wrong direction." I pick up Havi's spoon, scoop a little cottage cheese onto it, and put it into her right hand. She curls her fingers around the spoon and slowly brings it to her mouth. A few curds make it in. The rest lands in her lap.

Havi's left hand rests on the table in a fist. She should be able to relax her hands by now. I look at her belly. It's plump and healthy looking. She's getting what she needs, I decide.

* * *

Matt and I are sitting in the neurologist's office, watching Dr. Codman examining our baby. Dr. Codman performs a battery of tests similar to Havi's early intervention evaluation. Havi reaches for a ball; she follows a squeaky toy. Dr. Codman pushes against her arms to test her strength. She pushes and pulls Havi's legs. She asks us about our families' medical histories.

"Myra and Matt," she says in a grave tone. "I'm afraid your daughter has Cerebral Palsy."

"*What?*" Matt bursts out.

The room blurs. My mind wants somewhere safe to go. I focus on Matt's face, my rock. Matt himself—looks destroyed.

Dr. Codman explains that a growing number of CP cases are genetically driven and not due to traumatic birth, the disease's more common cause. She orders an MRI and refers us to Dr. Srivastava , a neurogeneticist, to help us understand the CP diagnosis. "Once we have more information, I'll be able to give you a better sense of the degree of severity," she tells us. "The good news is, Cerebral Palsy is nonprogressive. Havi can have a long life."

Matt mumbles a thank-you. We rush out of the clinic and into our car. Once Havi is settled in, Matt collapses over the steering wheel, sobbing.

Instinctively I call my parents. Pushing the words *Cerebral Palsy* out of my mouth triggers my own tears. It doesn't help to hear their heart-broken voices. They raised three healthy children. Matt takes several deep breaths, blows his nose, and calls his. Matt and I were planning to go back to work after Havi's appointment. We both cancel our meetings and go home.

Reset. Again.

I find some comfort—or at least seek some comfort—in thinking about Havi's long life with CP. Matt soothes himself the way he does: with action. He makes a list of the doctors Havi will need to see and the types of therapists who can help her develop the most skills possible.

We are advised to meet with a financial planner. He tells us to make sure Havi will be taken care of after we die.

CHAPTER 4

Diagnosis Day

December 17, 2019. Havi is fifteen months old.

Matt and I are standing in the hallway in the Department of Neurology at Boston Children's Hospital. Havi is in my arms. We've ended up in Dr. Srivastava's office after a three-month meandering odyssey through neurology, orthopedics, early interventions of multiple flavors, and several pediatricians trying to understand why Havi has missed developmental milestones.

Dr. Srivastava opens his office door and welcomes us in. The purple sweater under his white coat catches my eye. Havi loves purple. Could this be a good sign? He shakes my hand, then Matt's. "Call me Dr. Sid," he says.

"I'm Myra. This is my daughter, Havi. And Matt, her father."

"Hi, Havi, I'm Dr. Sid," he says to her sweetly. Then he turns to me. "She's beautiful," he says. "Come in."

"Havi can sit on the floor," Dr. Sid says. "We're going to start with a check of her mental status."

Matt and I sink to the floor next to our daughter.

On the home screen of Dr. Sid's phone, face-up beside him, I see a photo of two smiling children. *Healthy children,* I think reflexively. *What a gift.*

The room is overheated and stuffy. Matt unzips his blue Patagonia jacket.

Dr. Sid places a hand on Havi's knee to calm her momentarily.

"Does she always startle?" Dr. Sid asks.

Matt and I look at each other, confused, and then at Dr. Sid. "I noticed that Havi startled when Matt unzipped his jacket," he says. Does she do that often?"

"For the past few months," I answer. "We asked Havi's pediatrician about it. She said it's probably sensitive hearing."

Dr. Sid scribbles a note on his yellow pad. "Havi, let's play." He pushes a wooden box full of variously shaped plastic blocks toward her.

Dr. Sid presses the yellow triangle, which lights up. "Havi?" he says. "Would you like to try?" She responds by reaching for the box, and I exhale a sigh of relief. But she doesn't push the yellow triangle. Maybe she's too sophisticated for this kind of game, I think.

While distracting her with his left hand, Dr. Sid shakes a small bell with his right. Havi doesn't turn toward it. Dr. Sid puts a small pile of blocks in front of her. Havi doesn't reach for them. Dr. Sid offers her a ball, rolls it in front of her. Havi doesn't track its motion.

Havi's movements have always been slow and smooth. I considered them deliberate and graceful. But this setting darkens my view. My chest feels tight. My insides are squeezed. I'm clutching the hope I've come here with: that Dr. Sid will tell us, *Everything's going to be fine.*

Eight minutes that feel like eight lifetimes later, Dr. Sid puts the toys away and looks directly at Matt and me. The two of us exhale in sync, our breaths echoing in the room.

"Well. I have some questions," Dr. Sid begins. "Were you tested for Tay-Sachs?" He begins listing indicators: the startle reflex, Havi's move-ments, the developmental delay. Matt and I both interrupt him. It couldn't be Tay-Sachs. We had learned about Tay-Sachs in Hebrew school as kids; it's a horrific disease, one that disproportionately affects Ashkenazi Jews, but we are a generation that benefits from screening and we had been tested two years earlier. "I'm a carrier, but Matt isn't," I try to reassure Dr. Sid. "She doesn't have Tay-Sachs."

"I'd like to give Havi a blood test during Monday's MRI to be sure. And Myra," he adds, gesturing toward my pregnant belly, "you need to see a high-risk obstetrician immediately for a test on the fetus. Just to be safe."

* * *

Monday arrives quickly. I haven't slept well for the handful of nights since the appointment with Dr. Sid. We wake Havi up early and get her into the car with her pajamas on. Her MRI is the first one scheduled that Monday morning. My mom had flown in from Philadelphia to support us. It felt good to tell Havi, "Grandi is here with us."

Matt, Havi, and I, along with my mom, arrive thirty minutes early for Havi's MRI. The four of us sit in the quiet waiting room staring at the fluorescent fish painted on the walls. After an hour, Matt gets up and asks the receptionist about the delay. I look down at Havi, relaxing in my lap. She smiles at me, her eyes big and bright. I feel a burst of hope.

"Havi Goldstein!" the nurse finally calls out. She leads Havi, Matt, and me into a small, curtained-off exam room. My mom stays in the waiting room.

Prepping Havi for the MRI, the nurse struggles to insert an IV line into a vein in her tiny hand. By the time the nurse succeeds, Havi's hand is bruised and bleeding. "I can only let one of you into the MRI," the nurse says, looking from Matt to me and back again. "You go," I tell Matt. He's the doctor. And I hate needles.

Ten minutes later I look up from my chair in the waiting room to see the nurse leading a weeping Matt to me. He sags into my arms, burying his head in my hair. When he can speak, Matt tells me that Havi let out a little cry as they injected the drugs into her IV; then she went limp and unconscious in his arms. When he put Havi down on the bed and saw her lying there unresponsive, he burst into tears.

* * *

That afternoon, after the MRI is over and Matt has dropped Grandi and Havi and me off at home, he drives back to Boston Children's to pick up a blood test kit from Dr. Sid, who has asked us to give blood so that they can run a bunch of other tests to help figure out what Havi might have. I jump on a work call, pretending that life as I know it has been uninterrupted. When Matt gets home I am in our bedroom, talking to a colleague about a presentation I had missed. As soon as I see his pale face, I hang up the phone. Matt starts to talk in his serious voice—low and soft—and uses some medical jargon. As I try hard to listen, my legs turn into bricks and our room starts to spin. All I hear is:

"Dr. Sid showed me an image of Havi's MRI and pointed to several areas of her brain. He said that these types of images are characteristic for Tay-Sachs disease. 'I am so sorry,' he said."

As he says the words *Tay-Sachs*, I scream.

I barely process the things Matt says next: *No cure. Rare. Destroys the nerve cells in the brain and spinal cord. The symptoms progress until they lead to death between two years and four years old.*

CHAPTER 5

Shabbirthday

December 18, 2019.
Twenty-four hours ago, Matt and I walked out of the hospital with Havi in our arms, having just been told that she will die. Now we're walking back in, for the test—called the chorionic villus sampling—that will tell us whether the baby I've been carrying for eleven weeks will also die of Tay-Sachs disease.

This is the last place I want to be. I don't have to ask to know that Matt feels the same way.

We park in the familiar lot at 75 Francis Street and walk through the hospital's front door. The chaos of the lobby is a blur that can't compete with the clanging thoughts in my head. We ride the elevator to the third floor, follow the signs to the high-risk obstetrics clinic. A young woman calls us as soon as we're settled into the waiting room and introduces herself as Melissa, our genetic counselor. She leads us into her office and nods Matt and me into soft, matching armchairs. A moment later we're joined by Dr. Samantha Grant, my new obstetrician.

My body relaxes a bit. I can see Matt relaxing, too. I sense that I'm in a safe place and in trustworthy hands. Melissa and Dr. Grant ask how we are and listen intently as we stumble through describing our overturned lives. They explain what the next few hours are going to look like. The procedure itself is extremely safe, they say, and will last only a few minutes. You'll feel fine afterwards.

Melissa walks us down the hall and into a dimly lit exam room. Waiting in the room is a team of doctors: my new OB, two residents, and a senior attending. I wonder if I've now become one of those fascinating teaching cases that Matt used to talk about when he was in residency.

I climb up onto the hospital bed and pull up my shirt to expose my belly. A fuzzy ultrasound image of my uterus snaps into view on the screen mounted to the wall. The sensation of the ultrasound probe is different from when I was pregnant with Havi. This time I feel fear, not excitement.

"I'm going to insert a needle into the womb," Dr. Grant says. "I'll guide it to the placenta using the image on the ultrasound scan, then take a sample of cells from the placental tissue. Please let me know if you feel any pain at all." Matt holds my hand. I lie back, and within minutes, it's done. "Everything went great," Dr. Grant says, helping me sit up. "We'll know the results in three or four weeks. But we'll have you back in before then for a more in-depth conversation about your options based on these results. Any questions?"

How do we live like this? I want to answer. But I don't. Matt and I walk back to our car in silence, hand-in-hand.

As Matt steers the car onto the Jamaica Plain Parkway, I'm relieved to let the hospital complex disappear from our view. Tall birch and oak trees line the road, their leafless limbs making this winter day feel even colder. I reach beneath my sweater to trace the small bandage on my lower abdomen. Three to four weeks of holding my breath, taking care of our dying daughter, wondering if I'll have to face the decision to abort my second child.

Matt startles me, banging his fist against the steering wheel, staring at the road with tears streaming down his cheeks.

"How do we do this? How do we watch our daughter die?" he weeps. I reach over and put my hand on his thigh.

"I know," I whisper. How can this be? How can I be sitting in this car with my husband, driving home from the hospital, in this terrifying situation? As we drive past the pond, the baseball diamond, the grassy field where kids play soccer in the spring, I close my eyes and see a movie of the future we'll never know. We'll never see Havi's first steps. Never hear her say *Mamma* or *Dadda*. Never watch her play on that grassy field or make friends or get on the school bus. We'll never help her with her algebra homework, or take her to dance class, or…

I open my eyes, but the movie won't stop. I feel foggy and disconnected. Life—my life, her life, our life as we'd planned it, with its moments and milestones, is collapsing in space.

I pull my knees up to my chest and rest my head on my knees. Out of the corner of my eye I see Matt's hand gripping the steering wheel so hard, his knuckles are white. His anguished question hangs in the silence between us.

"I don't know, M. I don't know." As I'm fighting tears, something shifts in me. Somehow, suddenly, I do know. "I know what we'll do," I say. "We'll celebrate the shit out of her. We'll squeeze every ounce of beauty and love into her for as long as we can."

Matt looks over at me with wet eyes. I keep going, through the knot the size of a golf ball in my throat.

"Every Friday night." I'm winging it, picking up speed as I go. "We'll celebrate every Shabbat. Like it's Havi's birthday. We'll celebrate all the birthdays she would've had. We'll invite our people."

"Like a combination of Shabbat and birthday?" Matt glances over at me. "A ... Shabbirthday?!"

I smile. It hurts.

"That's good. A Shabbirthday," I say. "That's how we'll do this. From one Shabbirthday to the next."

* * *

Three days after learning that Havi has only a year or so to live, we celebrate her first Shabbirthday. A dozen of her aunts, uncles, grandparents, and close friends descend on our home. No one pretends the heartache isn't there. Havi is showered with gifts: a onesie; cake and balloons; a plush toy avocado, a warm challah; an elegant gray dress with white leggings—her first Shabbirthday outfit. Havi eats two helpings of sweet potatoes and giggles her way through the extra frosting that Matt feeds her with his finger. Her body vibrates in her seat; she kicks her legs with excitement.

Our home feels full and warm. Everyone here is full and warm, nestling together in the flickering light of the Shabbat candles, and the reality of Havi's terminal illness. None of us masks our pain with fake smiles. None of us hides from the joy and laughter that bubble up from our deepest, most pain-filled inner selves. Havi spends every moment in the arms or the lap of someone who loves her.

By 10:00 p.m., our loved ones have gone home. Havi is asleep. Matt and I sit down to write about the night.

Since that first Shabbirthday, we celebrate Havi that way every Friday night, no matter what we're doing or where we are; no matter what's happening in the world or in our lives. Each week we invite friends and family for good food, wine, and of course, ice cream for dessert. We listen to music, dance, and read poetry. When everyone goes home, Matt and I write a letter to Havi describing the evening we just shared. Every Saturday morning, we post that letter on CaringBridge, sharing news of Havi and the transformative and painful life lessons we're learning as we accompany her through her life.

* * *

"Go see a rabbi," people respond when we tell them about Havi's diagnosis and prognosis, and they don't know what else to do or say. We decide to take their advice. In January 2020, we arrange for a meeting with Rabbi Rachel, a Boston rabbi who comes highly recommended. Technically, we're members of this rabbi's synagogue. Before we knew Havi would never attend school, we'd applied to the preschool there; when Havi was a newborn, we'd attended the kids' High Holy Days services.

Rabbi Rachel greets us warmly and leads us into her office. "I'm so glad you could be here," she says. "And where is your daughter?"

"Havi stayed at home with her grandparents and aunts and uncles," I answer. "She's in the best hands."

"I'm relieved you two are getting out of the house on your own. That's a very good sign."

A good sign of what, I wonder. But I don't question the rabbi.

The rabbi's assistant brings us coffee in small Styrofoam cups. It's weak and tasteless, but warm. Matt and I sit on the couch facing her in a beautiful office filled with antiques and books and Judaica.

"Please," she says, "tell me your story."

The rabbi listens quietly and with evident compassion. I feel comforted by her presence. I'm hoping—expecting—that she'll become a guiding presence for us. She recommends that we read *When Bad Things Happen to Good People* by Rabbi Harold Kushner, and I make a mental note to order a copy.

I tell her about turning our Shabbats into weekly celebrations of Havi. "We call them Shabbirthdays," I say, with the first actual enthusiasm I've felt since the diagnosis.

Abruptly the rabbi leans forward, shifting her body from relaxed to upright. "I wouldn't commit to anything like that," she says matter-of-factly.

Shocked, I meet her eyes. They seem to have lost their warmth.

"You don't know how you're going to feel two weeks from now," she says stiffly. "And think about when she is gone, how hard your Fridays are going to feel. If I were you..."

But you're not us, I think, a hot spot of anger sparking in my belly. "...I'd live your lives the way you always have. And take a lot of photos."

A half hour later, Matt and I drive home along the Jamaica Plain Parkway through Jamaica Plain, now our thoroughfare for difficult conversations. "That was bullshit," I blurt.

Matt has sunken down so low in the driver's seat, the steering wheel looks too far from him to hold. "I can't believe she said that," he agrees.

"We're all in on Shabbirthdays," I declare. "And I wish she had used Havi's name."

CHAPTER 6

The Mistake

I am reeling from our visit with the rabbi. I counted on the time with her for guidance and stability in the wake of the worst possible ending. And then it was anything but that. And, the reality of Havi's impending death is settling into my bones. Needless to say, we are not sleeping well. One night, I stir in my sleep and turn toward Matt's side of the bed, reaching out for him, only to feel cold sheets against my hand. He is up again. It is quiet and the room is dark. I sense it is the middle of the night. Matt has never been a particularly good sleeper, and these last few weeks have only made that worse.

I slide out of bed and walk slowly into the hallway. I can see a blue glow down the hall and walk toward it: Matt sits on the living room couch with his laptop on his knees. He looks like he had during residency—wearing scrubs, shirtless, his hair messed up from restless sleep.

"What are you doing up, Emmy? I wish you'd try to sleep." He doesn't look up from his screen. "Look at this," he continues, placing his two hands over his open mouth.

I sit down on the couch next to him and he turns the laptop screen toward me. It takes me a moment to orient myself. I had actually been sleeping deeply, which is so rare during these weeks that I had come to dread nighttime. It is in the dark and quiet when my mind goes to the scariest places. I lean toward the screen.

Matt's web browser is open to the patient portal at his primary care physician's practice. He is looking at an old message exchange with his doctor. "I started to think that somehow, maybe Havi's diagnosis was my fault. Like I had misremembered something, but look," he says.

He turns up the screen's brightness, so it glows like a beacon in the dark living room. I read through it quickly and then my eyes return to the first line and scan back and forth.

Test Results
To: Matthew Goldstein
From: James Turner, MD
Received:10/25/2017 10:21 PM EDT
Note:
Matt,

Your Tay-Sachs genetic testing came back today and was negative! Just seeing these now (at 10PM) otherwise would have called you to share the news!

I'm so sorry again about the unnecessary worry with the enzymatic test.

Looks like you're on my schedule in a few weeks so look forward to seeing you then.

Dr. Turner

"I am so sorry about the unnecessary worry," Matt repeats five times. "Are you? Are you sorry? How does this happen?!"

I sit there, stunned, tasting my tears as they fall into my mouth. Matt jams his fingers into his hair and squeezes them into a fist. The muscle on his forearm tightens.

"What does this mean?" I say. "Dr. Sid said you are a carrier based on the new bloodwork. I just assumed there was a spontaneous mutation or something."

"No, no. Not a spontaneous mutation. They made a mistake. They must have. I've been a carrier this whole time." Matt slumps back against the couch and stares off into the dark room.

Just then Havi's cry echoes down the hall.

"Should we go take care of her?" I gently place my hand on Matt's thigh.

His face is blank. I can see he is deep in a mess of thoughts, trying to understand how we had gotten here.

"Love, do you hear her?" I say. "Should we go?"

Matt closes his laptop.

"Yeah. Let's just bring her in the bed with us tonight."

* * *

The next day, we sit on the edge of our bed and Matt puts the phone on speaker. Over the previous forty-eight hours, he has poured over scientific literature on Tay-Sachs, spoken to world-renowned scientists in the field, and exchanged notes with company executives who are focused on rare pediatric diseases. He'd done all this to understand what our therapeutic options are for Havi.

This morning, Matt is on the phone with a colleague with whom he had, by sheer coincidence, taught a class with at Massachusetts General Hospital and who is one of the physicians leading a trial for gene therapy in Tay-Sachs. Matt wants to understand the therapeutic landscape for Tay-Sachs. And given his background as an MD-PhD with an expertise in the testing and development of new medicines in clinical trials, he speaks this language better than anyone.

We are the patients now, though. What a nightmare.

I can't follow all the details of the call, but I get the gist. It isn't good. I wait for Matt to finish the call before asking questions. He hangs up the phone and then stands up and begins pacing back and forth along the foot of our bed.

"I fucking hate this. It's so unfair." He bangs his fist against the bedroom wall beside the window.

"Is this worth pursuing?" I ask. "It doesn't sound like it is, but can you tell me what you heard?"

"Well, they'd need to do a neurosurgical procedure to administer the therapy. So, brain surgery. Havi would have to be on immunosuppressant drugs. She, and we, would be visiting the hospital regularly for scans of her brain, laboratory tests, and functional assessments."

"Okay, and there is no way to fix the enzyme? How can that be? It's just one enzyme. I don't understand."

"Well, the hope of gene therapy is that you can replace the bad or abnormal copy of the gene with a normal copy. But there's a lot of issues with that—surgery, immune suppression, etc. There are mutations in the DNA that encode the enzyme. Those mutations result in an enzyme that cannot function normally, and in some cases, cannot function at all."

"Okay. So what do we know, with any kind of certainty?"

"We know there are only two children with infantile Tay-Sachs who have been treated in the world and we don't yet know how the trial impacted their disease," Matt says. "We know there is a chance that the therapy *could* prolong Havi's life. We don't know by how much."

"Prolong, okay. But what about enhance?"

"We know there may be a slowing of progression of the disease. And we know it isn't going to reverse the disease. Or cure her," Matt says. "She will still lose everything. And she will still die, relatively soon."

We both collapse onto the bed and hold each other. We must soon doze off to sleep for several hours because we awake a while later to a knock on the door. It is Tia, holding Havi. Tia has to leave for the day. We pop up from the bed. Tia gives Havi a big kiss and gently hands her to me.

CHAPTER 7

Charlie and Blyth

December 29, 2019. Havi is fifteen months old.

Matt and I sit on either side of Havi at the kitchen table, watching her eat blueberries and eggs. Between bites, she puts her hand on Matt's. She sneezes. A deluge of eggs lands on his arm. He laughs. She laughs. Real laughter. I adjust Havi's purple beanie and kiss her cheek. "It's nice to hear you laugh again," I tell Matt.

"Her laugh is the most intoxicating thing. How could I not laugh with her? Even though it hurts so much."

One of the symptoms of my shock and grief is isolation. Each time I tell someone what's happening with Havi, the truth of it becomes more real, and more unbearable. Also, even our best-intentioned friends and family members are prone to saying things that hurt, like "Maybe this is happening for a reason." At the same time, isolation is not the medicine I need, and I know it. So I force myself to reach out to those I trust, or at least to respond to them when they reach out to me.

So I take the call that comes in from my colleague, Rosemary. I step outside and stand on our front stoop in the cold, looking at the bare trees in the field across the street, talking with Rosemary about tomorrow's meeting of our organization's board of directors, where I'm scheduled to present the next year's strategic plan. For eighteen months I've been leading the nonprofit SquashBusters, Inc., a sports-based youth development program. I love my job, and I'm proud of SquashBusters' progress, giving our students chances to pursue their passions and purposes.

As we're talking, I realize I need to ask Rosemary to stand in for me. I'm in no state to do what needs to be done tomorrow. Suddenly, none of this important work matters to me. It has disappeared into another dimension, a dimension I can't reach, a dimension filled with all the things I used to care about that now seem trivial.

"Havi has Tay-Sachs," I blurt out. "We just found out. We're going to lose her in the next year or so. I can't be there tomorrow. I'm really sorry."

"Oh my gosh," Rosemary gasps. "I'm shattered for you. Of course I'll handle the presentation. And ... I have someone you need to meet."

I'm stunned. Someone I *need* to meet? The only thing I *need* is to be with my dying daughter. Why is Rosemary playing matchmaker? I barely got the words "Tay-Sachs" out of my mouth without choking on them. My world is about Havi and Matt now. I don't want to talk to a single other human being.

"I promise you'll understand why, once you meet my friend Blyth and her husband, Charlie," Rosemary goes on. "Do not spend another second thinking about the board report. Go be with Matt and Havi. I love you and I'm here."

"Thanks, talk soon." I hang up abruptly.

A few days later, I get an email from Blyth. I read it to Matt. "I am devastated on your behalf to learn that your little girl Havi has been diag-nosed with Tay-Sachs. That is just so very mean."

My anger at Rosemary evaporates. Somehow, I trust Blyth immedi-ately. She uses Havi's name and the words *devastated* and *so very mean*. She gets it. Maybe Rosemary was right to connect us after all.

Blyth and I exchange emails and make a plan to meet her and her husband, Charlie at their house in Newton, twelve minutes from ours. Still, I'm not sure if this is the right thing for us to do. What if they don't really, truly understand us?

Matt and I spend a few hours Googling Blyth and Charlie. We learn that they lost their daughter, Cameron, to Tay-Sachs nearly twenty years ago. After Cameron died, Blyth founded the nonprofit organization Courageous Parents Network (CPN) to support families like ours. Their mission: To empower, support, and equip families and providers car-ing for children with serious illness. Matt and I decide to meet them on Sunday afternoon, as planned.

As we get ready to go, Matt senses my lingering apprehension. "We don't have to stay very long," he says. "If it's not feeling okay, we'll just say we need to get Havi home for her nap."

"Thanks, love." How lucky am I, I ask myself for maybe the ten thousandth time, to have a sensitive and accommodating husband? We bundle Havi up in her purple jacket and matching purple hat and load her into the car seat. I sit in the backseat next to her, holding her hand, rubbing her calves, and shaking my water bottle. She loves that sound, and I love making her smile.

Charlie and Blyth's simple two-story house glows in the thin, wintry afternoon light. The lawn is blanketed in snow; lights shine warmly through the windows. *It looks cozy in there*, I think, despite my fears.

As we approach the front door, I smell wood smoke, which calms me even more. Havi is calm as I carry her. As always, she gives me strength. The door opens and there are Blyth and Charlie, and before we can even get inside, Charlie cups Havi's face with his two hands and gives her a gentle kiss on the forehead. "She is stunning. Those eyes. Oh my, the longest lashes," Blyth says.

Without another word, Blyth gives me and Havi the strongest hug. Charlie and Matt embrace. We switch places and hug again.

Blyth and Charlie are a good-looking couple, with a down-to-earth, chic, coastal aunt and uncle New England vibe. Charlie has bright blue eyes, and Blyth is effortlessly beautiful, with a warm, inviting smile. They're both in their fifties; their eldest daughter, Taylor, is about to graduate college and their youngest, Eliza, is heading to college this coming fall. They bring us into their kitchen, where we gather around a plate of homemade cookies and a pot of tea. They look into Havi's eyes in a way no one ever has before. I feel like they're seeing her as a precious, sacred being worthy of great adoration and love. I imagine they're seeing their own daughter, Cameron, in the way Havi's eyes follow the light. Blyth says Havi's blonde hair reminds her of Cameron's, the way it glimmers in the sunlight slanting through the kitchen window.

Blyth and Charlie know how to hold Havi so she can feel comfortable and relax. It's a relief to realize that, with them, I don't need to explain Havi's startle, her muscle spasms, how slowly she moves her arms, why she isn't speaking, why she coughs after eating a small amount of food, or that we aren't sure what she can hear. All of that—all the signs of Tay-Sachs—practically disappear at Blyth and Charlie's home with its crackling fire, and their honest, loving marriage; and an appreciation for long meals with plenty of wine. Our conversation leaps from spirituality to grief and love to changing family and friend dynamics. We waste zero time on small talk. We talk instead about what matters. How Matt and I can care for Havi and each other as we anticipate the unimaginable. How we want Havi at home or in beautiful places for the rest of her life—anywhere but the hospital.

We tell our new friends that we're exploring gene-therapy options but are unlikely to pursue an experimental trial. They validate our instincts. They made a similar choice twenty years ago. Instead of keeping Cameron in the hospital, they took a few days off every month and brought their girls to beautiful, quiet places.

"Twenty years ago, gene therapy wasn't an option. I don't envy the position you're in right now," Blyth says.

Charlie adds, "We learned to listen to Cameron. We would do it the same way again."

"No experimental trials," Blyth adds.

The two of them take the three of us on a tour of their home. The walls are lined with photographs of their three daughters. A feeling of gratitude spreads through my chest. I know we'll be able to talk with Blyth and Charlie about how to love and learn from our own dying daughter. They've already walked the narrow bridge between life and death, and they inhabit a *knowing* that makes me feel like I belong right here, with them. Between Havi's diagnosis and this moment, I haven't felt like I belong anywhere, except with Matt. It's been as if the world I knew had vanished. Everything felt unfamiliar and unsafe.

Charlie and Blyth see us as the couple we were before Havi's diagnosis, because they *were* us. Blyth says as much as we follow behind her on the house tour. "I can't stop looking at you, Myra. I was your exact age when this was happening to me."

The five of us settle in the living room near the warm fire. Blyth sits on the floor, her back against the couch, leaning on Charlie's legs. Matt and Havi and I sit on the other couch, facing them. Matt wraps his arm around my shoulder, and Havi sits upright on my lap, a cheese stick in her hand. Blyth and Charlie tell us all about Cameron, including how the only time in her life that she was ever really uncomfortable was one winter day when she wasn't dressed warmly enough. It hadn't gotten any worse than that. I breathe a sigh of relief, pulling Havi closer. I've been terrified that she'll be in pain. Now I relax a bit.

Blyth and Charlie talk to us about palliative care. Over and over, they say, Cameron had made it abundantly clear what she wanted. We hang onto every word as these two beautiful human beings share with us how they'd navigated, and were still navigating, their daughter's illness and death after nearly two decades. They talk, too, about their different grieving styles. Charlie had turned to meditation and contemplative practices. Blyth had weeded their yard of dandelions religiously. Charlie wanted to know exactly what was to be expected when their Tay-Sachs journey began. Blyth preferred to know less.

I feel soothed, hearing about Blyth and Charlie's nearly grown daughters, Taylor and Eliza. Both girls live rich, happy lives, fulfilling their own dreams. I see beauty and lightness, intertwined with tragedy, in Charlie and Blyth's lives. A tinge of envy seeps in. They have two healthy girls who know sisterhood. We have a dying daughter. And the future of our fetus is uncertain.

As Matt and I tell our story, we take turns holding and snuggling Havi on our laps. We tell our friends how much Havi loves food, a perfect fit with our habit of having long meals at the kitchen table. How she loves to laugh and erupts into unexpected giggles that change the course of a day. How her aunts, uncles, and grandparents from across the country have already descended on Boston. Along with other family members and friends who love Havi, we have formed an incredible posse.

"Havi's posse," Charlie says. He looks deep into our eyes.

"I love that." I can see, in Matt's eyes and body language, that he's instantly falling in love with Charlie.

Blyth and Charlie make it easy for us to be open to our fears and our broken hearts. It's dark when we tear ourselves apart. As we stand by the door sharing long goodbye embraces, Blyth and Charlie tell us that they'll be there for us as much or as little as we want. They'll follow our lead, they say. And they'll be checking in.

Matt and Havi and I pile into our car. As Matt drives toward the stop sign at the end of their street, we both look back at Blyth and Charlie's house. There they are, still standing in their doorway, waving goodbye as we drive away. We wave back. For the first time since the diagnosis, I think maybe we'll be okay. Maybe we can do this. Maybe life can still be beautiful. Maybe our marriage can become even stronger than it is.

Somewhere just beyond what our eyes can see, there's a great mystery unfolding in the world of the divine—a world that brought us together with Blyth and Charlie; a world I've never needed to recognize or appreciate the way I do now.

* * *

The drive home is quiet, until we're almost there. Matt catches my eye in the rearview mirror. "So, what do we do?" he asks me. I'm all too aware of what his question means.

Our first-born daughter has a fatal diagnosis. There is no known treatment that will save her life. How will we live while Havi is dying?

Both of us are struggling, Matt especially, with the medical system's approach to Havi's care. Our conversations with the provider team being assembled around Havi feel more like a directive than a choice. "You can do everything," the doctors keep telling us, "or you can do *nothing*." What parent wouldn't want to do "everything" for their child? Are we sociopaths to even consider other options?

Something Charlie and Blyth said keeps playing in my head: "Cameron made it so clear, over and over again, what she wanted and didn't want." Of course she did, and of course Havi will too. Havi has already been telling us. When she's happy to be outside, she turns her face to the sun and lifts her chin toward the sky. When she's squirmy or fussy, taking her outside calms her. Havi's giggles tell us that she loves being around most people. When she doesn't smile or engage with her eyes, I know she's not comfortable in someone's presence; maybe she's picking up on our tension, or theirs. We know she loves music because she kicks her feet when she hears it; we know she loves dancing in her Dad's arms because her feet beat against him when she does.

That night, after we get home, we sit with Havi in the quiet of her room, so we can really listen to her. We need to feel how she wants to live the rest of her life. I wonder if I'm a little crazy, believing I can listen to my child who can't talk. But my self-doubt evaporates as soon as I'm in her presence. The way we get information from Havi is difficult to explain, but it happens. I'd rather overestimate what I imagine to be Havi's messages than underestimate them. This experience has made me trust my maternal intuition. It's made me believe that the soul speaks.

Havi sits on Matt's lap, relaxing into the soft space between his shoulder and chest. I sit on the floor, massaging her feet.

"What do you think, peanut," Matt asks Havi, "about all this medical stuff? It might keep you with us longer. But if it does, it could be a lot for you to handle. We'll do anything—*anything* to have you be okay."

Listening to Matt, I realize he equates "okay" with "comfortable." So do I. It means that Havi will always be in the arms of someone who loves her, in the natural world as much as possible, and only in the company of people who get how sacred she is.

Matt continues talking Havi through the options. I watch in awe as he navigates this impossible conversation with tenderness and grace. My heart aches as much for him as it does for Havi.

Then Matt gets really quiet. We both sit very still, looking deeply into Havi's eyes, asking her in our hearts what she wants. It's amazing what happens when we shut out the noise—when we trust a look, a deep sigh, a slight shift, an extra nuzzle.

Matt and I look at each other.

"What are you hearing?" Matt asks me.

"What I'm hearing, and what I know, is that she hates the hospital," I say. "The loud noises make her startle. The bright lights bother her eyes. The needles hurt, the strangers she deals with don't get it. She doesn't want any of that. She just wants to be with us—and with her posse, her people."

"I get that too," Matt says. "I'm scared as hell, though. We do this on our own? No interventions, no experts?"

In that moment it's clear. We're going to take a different path, one that's neither "doing everything" nor "doing nothing." We're going to listen, watch, and follow Havi's lead.

I nod. "I think that's what we're going to do."

The two of us look at Havi, who's now fallen asleep in Matt's arms. She takes the deepest breath, with an extra sip of air at the top of a long inhale, and on her exhale, her face melts into the softest smile. Gently, Matt arranges Havi in her crib. We tiptoe out of her room, hoping, as we do every night, for a restful, uninterrupted few hours of sleep.

CHAPTER 8

Waiting and Justice

The next morning, we sit in the genetic counselor Melissa's small office with my new high-risk obstetrician, Dr. Grant. We are here for that in-depth conversation that Dr. Grant mentioned at the procedure. They have now reviewed the results from the Tay-Sachs re-testing that Dr. Sid ordered, and they have also reviewed our medical records. The results of the chorionic villus sampling on the baby growing inside of me won't be ready for another few weeks.

Melissa and Dr. Grant ask to see a photograph of Havi and express their deepest sympathies. I feel like they mean it, and I trust them. I see Matt's shoulders relax; I can tell he trusts them too.

Melissa explains Tay-Sachs disease and how it is inherited. She tells us that Tay-Sachs is caused by mutations in the gene for an enzyme called HexA that make that enzyme not function correctly. She explains how we each carry two copies of every gene and pass one of those two copies to our offspring. For a child to have Tay-Sachs, they must have two abnormal copies of the gene, one from each parent. Only one abnormal copy means you're a carrier. We know all of this but listen generously.

She then goes through our original test results, which had been obtained before I was even pregnant with Havi, when we underwent carrier screening for Tay-Sachs disease and a handful of other diseases that are common in the Ashkenazi Jewish population. She shows us my results, stating that I am a carrier, and then she shows us Matt's testing. The first test ordered is called an enzyme test, which looks at the function of the HexA enzyme. Melissa points to the numbers on the page: "Matt, this number means that you're a carrier."

Then she flips the page over and points again. "This is the test they ordered to confirm your carrier status—this was the wrong confirmatory test. You have a right to know, Matt, that a mistake was made." Matt nods quietly. His shoulders sag. "How could this be?" he whispers.

We sit in silence, waiting. Melissa speaks first. "I need to share some additional details about the chorionic villus sampling—is that okay to do now?" Matt and I both nod.

"We've put an order in for expedited results so I am hoping they come back to us at three weeks, not four. But it is impossible to guarantee that. Because we take a sample from the placenta, we can trust that the results will be accurate. I will call you as soon as I know. For now, I hate that you have to wait. Do you have any questions?"

"Is there anything we can do to get a quicker result? Myra will be fifteen weeks pregnant by the time we know. And three weeks is a long time."

"I am so sorry. I know. I promise this is the best we can do."

"Let's go Emmy, it's okay." I say. I want it to be okay.

* * *

We wait a long time in a crowded waiting room at Boston Children's Hospital before we are brought back to the small office where Havi's vision is tested. When the doctor finally enters the room, with a resident following her, she immediately launches into a description of what they had seen—the characteristic cherry-red spot that is a typical finding in kids with Tay-Sachs disease. She tells us that Havi will eventually lose her vision and recommends that we schedule a follow-up appointment to monitor how things are going. No warmth. No mention of our reality. Just the cold, hard facts.

As we walk out of her office, Matt turns to me. "A follow-up appointment?!? For what? So that we can arrive fifteen minutes early for our scheduled appointment to wait for forty-five minutes in a crowded waiting room before seeing the doctor? So that we can be told that Havi's vision is getting worse or maybe gone altogether? I am astounded at how blind the doctor was in seeing, hearing, feeling what Havi needed, what we needed. She never even asked."

He reaches out his arms for Havi. I pass her to him gently.

"I'm sorry, Peanut," he tells her. "We won't put you through that again."

Carrying Havi, Matt walks ahead of me, slumped over. His posture has changed recently. I remember how, when Matt and I started dating, he'd stand up straight and walk proudly, and how he'd had so much hope and optimism, and such a strong commitment to the craft of medicine. Now, it seems, he is being beaten down by the very system that had brought us to Boston in the first place. It crushes me.

* * *

I check my phone incessantly, still awaiting a call from our genetic counselor about our growing fetus. Any day now. I am almost fifteen weeks pregnant, and still afraid to fully embrace my pregnancy because I know that the new life I am carrying inside me is threatened by Tay-Sachs. Over these past several weeks, I haven't known how to exist in my body. Aside from my immediate family, I haven't told anyone I am pregnant. Havi's diagnosis has shattered everything we'd imagined about this next phase of our life. We are *supposed* to have a healthy toddler and be excited about having another baby on the way. But now we have a dying daughter and a possibly precariously fated fetus. It is too much to hold. I barely look at my belly.

* * *

"I have some news," I say as we begin to share Havi's Tay-Sachs diagnosis with our closest friends and family members. "Oh my god, Myra," I hear back over and over again from the person at the other end of the phone. Eventually, they admit, "I cannot imagine." Then inevitably they ask, "But how could this have happened?" Even though it doesn't change Havi's diagnosis, or her fate, I feel a need to protect her and us, to make it clear that this isn't her fault. Or our fault. I reply, "A mistake was made during our preconception genetic testing. They said Matt wasn't a carrier, but he is." The person's gasp from the other end of the phone reverberates in my ear long after I finish the call.

On another phone call, with a family friend named Jay, his gasp is followed quickly by sharp words: "This should never happen, ever, not today, not in a country like the United States, not in a city like Boston, not in a medical system with such powerful technology and tools. Never. Never. Never. And this cannot ever happen again. The system has to know about this. It has to change. Whenever you are ready, I will help you. I am here for you both."

As we live with Havi's diagnosis and watch closely for the signs that her progressive disease is beginning to steal away her abilities, Matt and I return often to our conversation with Jay. The idea of a lawsuit feels like too much to manage for me. But, as we talk with a small group of Matt's colleagues and our close friends deeply familiar with the medical system, it becomes clear that a lawsuit, which Jay wholeheartedly supports, might be the best path to force the system to change.

On the one hand, it feels superficial and futile to consider litigation in the context of losing our daughter. There is no recourse. There is no cure. There is no amount of money or attention or apology that could possibly soften our pain. And yet, there is also something that feels wrong about inaction, about not participating in system-level change or improvement so that this never happens to another family. And advocating for Havi, making her life known within the medical system, feels like the only way to fully parent her. We'll never get to advocate for her in school or on a sports team; we'll never defend her from a childhood bully or commiserate with her after a breakup or a falling-out with a friend or tell her to keep her head up when she doesn't get a job she really wants. Telling her story and taking legal action is our platform for parenthood.

We lean on Jay to help us find the best lawyer to represent us, to represent Havi. And he does. We trust Jay, his legal expertise and his love for Havi. After meeting with the lawyer several times, we feel safe entrusting him with Havi's story too. We talk again with Jay and decide to move forward with a lawsuit. We share everything with him. This evening he writes us:

> I reread all three reports with tears in my eyes—and anger. They are impossible to read. I can't imagine what the two of you felt. I know you both know this: You both did everything you should have done—and more— sadly, three doctors did not—exhibiting a high level of negligence—and I am so, so sorry. It validates your reasons for bringing a lawsuit to help to prevent this from happening to any other families in the future. Thank you trusting me.
>
> We love and think about all of you every day.
>
> Jay

CHAPTER 9

Beginnings

Since Havi's diagnosis, the idea of walking out the door and leaving her at home every day, to return eight hours later, feels wrong on every level. And yet, for both Matt and me, this is new territory. We'd devoted ourselves to our respective vocations—mine in education and youth development, and Matt's in medicine and research. I am in my ninth year at SquashBusters, serving as the chief program officer, and while I hate the idea of taking time away from a place that I believe deeply in, I have the benefit of working alongside a uniquely compassionate and generous CEO in Greg and CFO in Rosemary. They had become mentors and confidants long before Havi was born. We trust each other. Matt had recently joined a new company focused on developing new cancer therapies only a few months before Havi was born, working for a CEO with an outsized sense of humanity and heart around the things that really matter.

We know we only have twelve to eighteen months left with our daughter. We want to choose her every day, to anchor every day in Havi and let the rest of the world fall away for a while. We draw up plans for a "Havimoon" to begin in January 2020, one month after her diagnosis day. We will take her everywhere until we can't anymore. "Now is the time" becomes our mantra. Both of our employers endorse a two-month paid leave of absence, from mid-January to mid-March, and reassure us that our jobs are secure. We are not to worry about anything other than soaking up time with our daughter. The unique privilege of this isn't lost on me and I only wish every employer operated this way. Memories, we will come to discover, are the only lifeline we have. If we can make as many beautiful memories as humanly possible, we can always revisit them. Memory requires presence of mind and heart.

It is an impossible concept to fully embrace. But one that I feel compelled to believe. We'll need to invite Havi into our daily life, after she is gone, through our memories with her; through the ways she exists in us while she is here; through the experiences we share; through the way she transforms our sense of being. So we have to create as many memories as we can. And the way we will hold them is to make sure we are fully present. We are with her. Not observing her.

We decide we will start the Havimoon on the Southern California Coast. Matt spent a few of his elementary school years in San Diego and wanted to make new memories with Havi there. He also wanted to share all of California with Havi and me, so we plan to road trip our way up the coast to the San Francisco Bay Area, where Matt had lived the majority of his life. And as we travel up the Coast, we will celebrate every Shabbirthday we spend out there.

* * *

On the morning of January 7, my cell phone rings. I am still in bed after a long night with Havi. Matt is up though, getting ready for the workday. The area code 617 flashes on my home screen—it is a Boston number. I grab my phone off the bedside table, jump out of bed, open the bathroom door, and show Matt the number.

"Are you good to do this now?" he asks, toothpaste foaming on his lips.

"I guess. When else?" I swipe to accept the call before it goes to voicemail. My heart is beating right out of my chest.

"Hi, Myra, it's Melissa, your genetic counselor from the Brigham. Is now an okay time to talk? Is Matt around?"

"Hi," I reply nervously. "Yes, we're both here."

I put Melissa on speaker and Matt and I both sit back down on the bed, upright against our reading pillows. The room is dark; we don't bother to pull up the shades or turn on the lights.

"Good news," Melissa says.

Matt and I take a deep breath for seemingly the first time since hearing her voice.

"The fetus is not affected by Tay-Sachs. The results were..."

I stop listening. Melissa continues on, sharing more details about the testing and answering Matt's questions. The two of them could communicate on a different level, given their medical training. Meanwhile, I have what I need. I feel badly that Matt has to play dad-doctor in these situations, but I also know that he takes pride and comfort in knowing that he speaks this language.

"Do you want to know the sex?" Melissa asks.

"Yes," I reply, looking over at Matt. Normally, Matt and I always give each other a chance to weigh in, but I need to know. I feel that we have too much uncertainty in our lives. When there is something we could know, without ambiguity, I want to know it. Control. A powerful and elusive thing. Matt smiles at me, acknowledging my impatience but loving me anyway.

"Havi will have a little sister." Melissa's voice is warm and cracking, as if she is tearing up.

"Wow. What a gift," I say. I can't get any other words out. Matt jumps in: "Thank you so much for the call, Melissa. And for all of your support."

"Your family is beautiful, and I wish things were so different. I'll be thinking of you all. Call if you need anything."

Matt presses the end-call button. "That is how all healthcare practitioners should communicate," Matt remarks. "She was so warm and clear. It all felt very personal in the best way." Even in this moment of personal intimacy, he couldn't help himself from weighing in on the system that failed us. I pace around our bedroom, and I start to brush my hair with a toothbrush. I'm rattled with emotion, and put the toothbrush down on my bedside table. I collapse under the sheets and touch my belly. It feels alive for the first time in this pregnancy. My mind moves to sisters and everything amazing I have known about them from the relationship with my own sister. And then my mind screams as I see the shattered dream for Havi's sister. I feel like I am living someone else's life. And yet we are going to have a healthy baby girl next summer. The pregnancy is viable. The baby isn't in danger. I have never experienced so many conflicting emotions at the same time: Relief, excitement, anguish, fear, dread, hope, and gratitude all form into the biggest lump in my throat. In this moment, I'm not sure if I'll ever be able to get out of bed.

PART
II

"Ritual is the antidote to helplessness."
SUKIE MILLER

CHAPTER 10

Havimoon

A few days later, on January 12, less than a month after her diagnosis, we wake Havi at an ungodly hour and drive to Boston's Logan Airport to whisk her away to Southern California. Havi has always been an amazing traveler, and this trip is no exception. Everywhere we take her, she is showered with compliments on how sweet and calm she is and how big and beautiful her eyes are.

We land in San Diego to clear blue skies and sunshine. We collect a truckload of luggage from baggage claim and make our way to the rental car center. "She is so well behaved." The person who helps us says, staring deeply into Havi's eyes. "How do you do it? I have three children. I can't get them to stay quiet for a minute. You're lucky." I want to throw up. "You have no idea. And we have no idea what we're doing," I reply.

We fill up an absurdly oversized SUV rental, and head for a cozy little inn in Del Mar. As soon as we get Havi in the stroller for a sunset jog along the beach, she closes her eyes and dozes peacefully. Just like us, Havi loves being near the ocean and in the sun—over and over again, it puts her at peace.

It doesn't take us long to get into a rhythm, and each of our long days by the sea is a dream. Every morning we wait patiently until we hear Havi stir in her crib and then fight over who gets to scoop her up. Her little body is always so warm, and she curls onto my shoulder and rests there for a moment as she lets her sleeping ebb away. Then she puts her little hands on my chest and pushes up, lifts her face to mine with her two bright eyes and a smile that melts my heart every time. Our mornings hold some of our sweetest moments. We goof around and play and watch the dawn light spread out over the soft morning waves.

For parents of healthy children, I imagine these moments as "extras" in a day filled with the main events. Not for us. And inevitably, at some point, Havi makes it abundantly clear that she is ready for breakfast. Then we race to the restaurant for blueberry pancakes or French toast, both of which she devours with vigor—sometimes eating so many pancakes that Matt and I feel a little nauseous for her. We usually follow Havi's mammoth breakfasts with a walk around town while she perfects the thirty-minute "snooze and rally" in the stroller, and then we are off and running for the rest of our day. We spend four wonderful days in Del Mar, where we run with Havi on the beach; hike in Torrey Pines State Reserve, one of the wildest stretches of land on the Southern California Coast; and eat delicious meals outside in the sunshine. Havi is happy in Del Mar.

Every day, we play her favorite songs in the car and dance together on the bluffs overlooking the sunset. My Havi song is Van Morrison's "Have I Told You Lately [that I love you]" and Matt's is Fleetwood Mac's "Landslide." Matt and I both cry whenever we sing these songs to her, but she always snuggles under our chins, as if urging us to finish.

Our days are full and Havi almost always starts to fall asleep during dinner, but she loves to be at the table with us and fights to stay awake. Most nights Matt and I crawl into bed just a few minutes after she—we decide that being in our dreams is better than being without her while she sleeps. "Sorry I lied about her age tonight at dinner. I just hated the way that waiter looked at her." I say to Matt just above a whisper. "I know, love. Me too. So, are we going with ten months?" "Seems right to me. How fucked up, though." Matt pulls me close. "Beyond."

After our fourth day in Del Mar, we pack up the SUV and head north along the coast to our next stop in Santa Monica. We time the trip to match Havi's morning nap routine, set our fresh-brewed coffees in the cupholders, turn on Charlie's Bela Fleck playlist, and drive into the misty, marine-layered morning. Charlie and Blyth listened to this same playlist during the last months of Cameron's life. Connecting with them through music is life sustaining—their enduring marriage, beautiful family, and full life come alive in the lyrics of the songs they'd chosen, and those lyrics nurture us. Charlie and Blyth are the first people to introduce us to the power of ritual in grief, an essential teaching in moving with it.

Rituals, both public and private, create opportunities to explore what is most vulnerable in us, and then enable us to share that vulnerability with others. Havi's posse evolved from such ritual sharing; and these friends and family who also carry Havi with them expand our access to

46

her. Our experience with the power of ritual personifies Francis Weller's observation that, "there are certain things that can happen only within the container of ritual, where the neglected, repressed parts of us are invited to speak."[1] And rituals, according to Charlie and Blyth, can be as simple as listening to a song that makes us laugh, cry, or remember. This becomes one of a handful of lessons, which, only in looking back, are Matt and I able to distill as such. We have actually intuited these lessons before we can even name them, but we become conscious of them over time.

About halfway through the playlist, thirty minutes into the drive, Havi breaks our peaceful journey with a crying spell that leaves her face tear-strewn and her eyes puffy. I give up my seat next to Matt, and crawl back to comfort her. In this moment, I'm frustrated with her. Why can't she fall asleep in the car like so many of my friends' kids? I hate myself for this thought.

For her fifth Shabbirthday, on January 17, she is once again showered with love. Her Aunt Maggie, Matt's sister, flies in with her three-month-old daughter Hannah from Colorado. I knew and loved Maggie before I fell in love with Matt. Maggie and I met during our freshmen year at Dartmouth College as soccer teammates and quickly grew so close. Maggie shared my passion for education and social justice, took me to Passover Seders at Dartmouth's Chabad Center, and encouraged me to have my first alcoholic drink at college. Now, it is wonderful and also heartbreaking to see her younger daughter, Hannah, because I can't help but think that Havi should have a lifetime to travel to beautiful places with her baby cousin. There is an urgency to the time they'd share during this visit because we don't know when or if they will spend time together again.

I also feel resentment, which I hate, but it is hard to be with healthy babies and toddlers. Impossible, really. But still, this is my niece. I know I love her and I can't fully give myself to her without being inauthentic, and most often I feel like a horrible aunt. Maggie has intentionally left Ayla, her older daughter, back at home in Colorado because that dynamic is even more painful. Ayla and Havi look alike, and at age two, Ayla walks and talks and picks out her clothes and brushes her hair and tells us she loves us and seems to grow and change every day. And anytime we talk

---

[1] Tim McKee, "Geography of Sorrow: Francis Weller on Navigating our Losses," *The Sun Magazine*, October 2015, 4–15.

with her on the phone, she asks for her cousin Havi. Ayla does all the things Havi never will, and while we know we love her, we can't handle seeing that. And our failure to handle it is devastating to both of us. Especially for Matt, who prides himself in being a devoted older brother.

At the very same time, there is much to celebrate, including the many cakes, cookies, and balloons that our family members and friends send, and little presents like an avocado-imprinted onesie. In fact, our incredible posse of family and friends keeps the hotel staff quite busy with all the packages being delivered. That Friday is a beautiful, warm day, particularly in contrast to the twelve-degree days we have left behind in Boston, so we take Havi swimming at the hotel pool before dinner. She squeals and giggles with delight in the water with Matt, kicking her legs effortlessly as if the water has the power to wash away Tay-Sachs.

With the sun setting on another Shabbirthday, it is hard to believe that a full month has passed since Havi's diagnosis. It had snowed on that brutal day, and the frothy flakes floating down belied the crushing weight that had been placed upon us. We can still feel that weight, but in California, Havi's smile and her energy and her joy in everything we do together gives us more than enough strength to move forward every day.

As we walk along the Santa Monica beach at sunset after dinner that night, though, I turn to Matt and tell him, with tears in my eyes, "I am afraid of Havi being alone wherever she has to go next. She's so good when she is with us. In our arms, snuggled against our chest. I am not sure I can do it. Let her go. You know?"

The idea of any kind of afterlife might have comforted me before, but not now, not as I imagine it for my daughter. I had found solace in the concept of heaven, but now, as Havi is about to be thrust from this earthly world prematurely and tragically, it becomes impossible to imagine a soft, safe, beautiful landing for her. I wonder if I've upset Matt because he walks silently. "I think there are lots of people to hold her on the other side." He finally says. I don't know.

I am not sure if Matt fully believes that, but it is what I need to hear him say in this moment, and I am grateful. As we walk along the beach, we take turns convincing ourselves and each other that there is more to this life than what we can see and feel around us. And that, we agree, is a good thing because to not believe—or not try to believe—in an afterlife means giving up on having an eternal relationship with our daughter.

After a while, we grow quiet, and I decide I don't have to consider those painful things any longer—not while I can still reach into Havi's stroller and stroke her soft cheeks. Instead, in this moment, I vow to take even better care of her, to brush her teeth more regularly. As she smiles up at me, I notice that her teeth are looking a tiny bit yellow from where I stand, probably because she'd recently discovered apple juice. I notice the sky. It is purple.

CHAPTER 11

On the Road

After a week in Los Angeles, we leave to drive up the Pacific Coast. Matt and I had once spent a few nights in the Ojai Mountains, and we are excited to share that magical place with Havi. On the drive up, Havi snoozes, resting up for our next adventure. Matt and I talk about her the whole way—laughing and crying and taking turns reassuring each other that we'll be okay. As we talk, Havi occasionally sighs or yawns or makes some other little sleepy sound, and we take deep breaths and feel better knowing she is right behind us.

We arrive in Ojai, a small, picturesque city nestled in a valley, just as the afternoon is turning to evening, and walk the beautiful hills as the day cools and the sky turns pink. Ojai's days are warm and sunny and its evenings cool and crisp, and we fall right back into our Havi rhythm and relish another delicious week together.

We spend our mornings warming up by the fireplace in our room and playing with Havi until it is time for breakfast. Our version of play with Havi consists of slow dancing, snuggling under all the covers, sitting on every piece of hotel furniture, rubbing lotion gently on her body, and massaging her feet to prepare for the day. For the most part, we continue Havi's ultimate breakfast experience, though one morning, when we chose to lay off the blueberry pancakes and switch to eggs, Havi lets us know that she has strong dietary preferences. She is grumpy the rest of the morning. "Point taken, Havi girl," we tell her. "Blueberry pancakes from now on!" I consider the tragic humor in not needing to care about things like a balanced meal.

We spend the better part of the rest of each day outdoors in the sunshine. We take Havi to the hotel pool three days in a row and she continues to love being in the water. I have a sneaking suspicion that part of why she loves the pool is because Matt holds her, sings to her, and waltzes through the water with her as his dancing partner. We always make sure to go to the pool at a time of day when we have it all to ourselves. That way Havi can kick and squeal and sing to her heart's content, and I avoid seeing other kids. I hate the fact that I can't be around other kids, but I really can't bear seeing healthy, thriving toddlers playing. It is too painful.

We find some beautiful hiking trails nearby in Los Padres National Park. Seated up above Matt's shoulders, strapped in a heavy-duty hiking backpack, Havi takes in the spectacular views of the valley and the ocean beyond. I am almost five months pregnant by now, so Matt carries Havi nearly the entire way. I resent the fact that I can't do it but she loves to play with Matt's hair anyway, and strokes his back as he walks, smiling and cooing and looking around, ever so observant and curious about the sights and sounds all around her.

On one hike in the foothills around Ojai, we walk through a grove of Pixie tangerines, small orange globes that hang by the hundreds from the trees around us. A sign reads "NO PICKING." Matt reaches up and picks one anyway—he holds it over his shoulder to show Hav, who sits in the carrier on his back. She giggles—whenever she laughs, we have to as well. Havi can't speak but we never struggle to understand how she feels. I write that night in our journal:

> You talk in smiles—perhaps the most instinctive, simple, and powerful form of communication. We have full conversations as you make your way through all the smiles of the world. You tilt your head back and let out an open-mouthed smile and we know you couldn't be happier.... Then there are your closed-lip smile, your flirtatious smile, your guilty smile, and your lopsided smile. With each one you make us feel like you're just seeing us for the first time, like you're so excited to be with us again. Your eyes sparkle and you stare deeply into our souls. Sometimes we have to look away as we wipe tears from our cheeks because you've moved us so deeply with your simple smile and twinkly eyes. Speaking of smiles, we know that one of the "functions" you'll lose is the ability to smile. Dad and I talked about this over pizza dinner the other night. Dad asked me if that was the thing I was most scared of. "I'm scared of it all," I said, and Dad agreed.

We are learning to live alongside grief, appreciating its power to keep us close to Havi. We're learning that pain and love can coexist. While we risk our hearts, we're expanding them too. Every week, one of us is lead writer, and the other "editor" for our Saturday morning postings on CaringBridge. Often, after I read Matt's entry, I feel even closer to him. Many times, I discover that I haven't realized where his grief was or what part of a day or moment of a day had been especially difficult for him. His postings give me a window into his heart and soul, and I find myself craving his living voice in these entries. I am blown away by his capacity to express himself, to lay bare his emotions, and even to make me laugh.

* * *

After a few sacred days in Ojai, we head further north to celebrate Havi's sixth Shabbirthday in Carmel, where we meet the rest of Havi's aunts and uncles: Uncle Jacob and Aunt Erin, Aunt Leah and Uncle Mike—all of whom we fondly refer to as the "Sibs." Jacob, my older brother, had an adjoining bedroom to mine growing up. The door was open unless something had gone terribly wrong in the world of pick-up sports. Jacob made me feel bold and capable—he used to pick me first in neighbor-hood games with his mostly older, male friends, and celebrated me every chance he got. He has always been my secret weapon because he puts me at ease, makes me laugh, and believes in me. While I always looked up to my older brother, in adulthood I've grown to admire the way he moves through the world with a mixture of ambition, authenticity, and kindness.

Jacob married Erin, who I met during my junior year at Dartmouth when she arrived as a freshman from California. We trained and stud-ied together—she is a talented athlete and an unflinchingly hard worker. Off the field, we could talk about everything and were inseperable. Erin is quietly brilliant, thoughtful beyond measure, and everyone's advocate. She always felt like home. Then Jacob fell for her.

Leah, my younger sister, turned many of the traditional older sister/ young sister dynamics on their heads. She always knew the right thing to say. Some nights, Leah would crawl into my twin bed to cuddle and talk before taking the short, eight-foot walk down the hall to her bedroom; I hoped I could absorb all of her wisdom and calm. After a middle school dance where I played matchmaker, but left with my own broken heart, Leah whispered: "It's okay, My-My. Those dances are kind of stupid. No one really is with the person they want to be with, I'm sure. It's all kind of fake." She was the best combination of everything: effortlessly beautiful, smart, and fun. She had a way of making me feel like I was a real-life hero or something. Being Leah's older sister has always been a generative force of good for me.

Then Leah fell in love with a boy, Mike, at Kenyon College, her freshman year. Mike, a smart and committed litigation lawyer, with an infectious laugh and disarming warmth, is excited and optimistic about even the littlest things, like the newest review on Wirecutter for toilet paper or dish soap. And in the way Leah always steadied me, I see that Mike has become that same steadying force for her. At six feet, four inches tall, Mike has become the gentle giant of our family.

With the Sibs awaiting us at our next destination the time passes quickly on the road. We have a call scheduled with our lawyer during our long drive up the California coast, and when it comes through, we are just north of San Diego, so we pull off Highway 1 into a beachside parking lot. We had hoped to take the call from the car, ideally during one of Havi's naps, but there we are, pulling over in a parking lot where people are closing up a small flea market and packing up their stalls. Havi is crying hard, so I walk her around the parking lot in the salty air while Matt gets on the phone with Rick, a Philadelphia-based lawyer who has come to us highly recommended by Jay. The fact that Rick is in Philly makes me feel more relaxed with him, and the moment we meet him, we feel like he has the compassion and ferocity to be our best advocate.

As I roll the stroller back and forth past the car, I watch Matt intently, trying to get a sense of how the call is going. He gestures a lot with his hands, but then he stops abruptly and tilts his head back. Finally, he ends the call and gets out of the car. Havi is asleep by now and we know she'd startle if we try to transfer her back to her car seat, so we continue to walk together.

"How'd it go? What did he say?"

"It was fine," Matt replies. "We obviously have a strong case. But they are going to do everything to use the fact that I'm a doctor against us."

"What does that even mean? Actually, don't answer that. It makes me want to puke."

I clench my fists and look at the waves in the distance. "I already hate this case," I say. "If it's going to take even an ounce of energy away from Havi, we should just stop right now. Really, let's just stop."

We come to a bench and sit down. Matt puts one hand on my back and moves the stroller back and forth with his other arm. "No, no," he says. "That call should be it for a while. They have everything they need. We won't need to do much of anything until the deposition."

* * *

We arrive at our hotel to find a room fully stocked with all of Havi's necessary foods: string cheese, blueberries, avocados, and graham crackers. The Sibs had worked their magic. We had been in Carmel once before too, when I was pregnant with Havi, for Jacob and Erin's wedding. Now we are staying at the place where Jacob and Erin had held their rehearsal dinner, where Havi had listened in utero to her dad's and Leah's toasts given on that holy night.

It feels so right to be back in this place with everybody. Erin and Jacob are living on the West Coast now, and for this Shabbirthday, Erin brings a challah all the way from a bakery in Woodside, California, which she and Jacob had picked up on their drive down to meet us. The Sibs keep on showing up for us and Havi in all sorts of small, meaningful ways, which makes being around them feel like everything is going to be okay—and that is the biggest gift imaginable. Showing up—in the everyday moments. Not the ones with formal invitations, but the ones that require us to be enmeshed in each other's lives. These are the moments that create relationships that last.

The next morning, we make our final push north, leaving Carmel for the San Francisco Bay Area and Matt's childhood home where Grandma and Grandpa were eagerly awaiting Havi's visit. There we would meet Tia and her thirteen-year-old daughter Vicel, who would fly in from Boston, and we would make sure they get a taste of the Havimoon. Matt is excited to bring Havi to all of his favorite eating spots, running spots, and beautiful places. He writes his weekly letter to Havi after one of our hikes:

Dear Peanut,

We hiked through Tennessee Valley to where the hills split and the trees gave way to small, crunchy, beachy shrubs. The path curved around a bend and into the sunlight and the black sand beach twinkled in the morning sun. I think you knew we were close to the ocean. A small stream wound across the sand and we tiptoed our way across the bigger rocks to get to the edge of the waves. Your hair bounced in the wind and you opened your mouth and rocked your head back and forth to taste the air. You love the wind—maybe it's the feeling of it on your face or the smells of the earth and the water. Whatever it is, you kick your legs, and coo, and get all excited whenever it blows around us.

As we squatted on the sand, I heard laughter from somewhere over my shoulder and I turned to see a little girl streaking toward the waves, her shoes kicked off and her hair streaming back behind her. Maybe she was five or six years old. For a moment I imagined you doing that one day—on another beautiful, sunny day in January in the future—with me and Mom walking somewhere behind you. I even smiled a little, thinking of it. And then I remembered why we were standing on that warm beach in the middle of January. Because we are going to lose you eventually. These things are both beautiful and hard for us, Peanut.

I love you,

Dad

* * *

Later this week, on January 30, we celebrate Jacob's birthday with an early dinner: 4:30 p.m. has become the new 7:00 p.m., and we actually love it. Havi has breakfast for dinner (cheesy scrambled eggs) and smiles and laughs along with everyone else. The eggs have enough butter and cheese to satisfy her. She sits on Jacob's lap when the birthday cake arrives and helps him blow out a single candle.

As I cut the cake into slices, Jacob bends down to sniff the scent of

Havi's hair and his eyes get wet; he looks over at me and we share a beautiful and painful moment of our devastating reality: that Havi will never blow out her birthday candles, never experience a birthday party the way kids should, never stick her face in a cake or eat too much ice cream. The *nevers* quickly pile up in my mind. But then Havi smiles, wraps her little finger around Jacob's, and brings us back to the present, back to our brimming table.

Havi's seventh Shabbirthday at Grandma and Grandpa's is as balloon-and-challah-and-love-filled as always. But it also marks the end of our Havimoon. We have tickets to fly back to Boston the next day.

As we repack our suitcases that night after dinner, just as the dread of returning to our reality creeps in, we get an email from Charlie, who reminds us that the Havimoon is a mindset. We have to learn to let go of the physical manifestations of this experience and let in its most profound and ever-lasting essence. This is our new challenge. It gives me a sense of peace as I fall asleep that night, even knowing we are saying goodbye to the beautiful West Coast sunsets and our time there.

CHAPTER 12

Life's Arc

Tia picks us up from the airport, which softens the hard landing and buffets the low thirty-degree temperatures and wintery mix that greet us in Boston. She carries a balloon with her and scoops Havi right up. The two of them giggle in the backseat during the car ride home. Matt and I sit in the front, smiling and squeezing each other's hands, knowing Havi will never know anything but the utmost love.

On our first night back home, Matt and I sit with Havi at our kitchen table, staring at each other, until late. We have a hard time getting Havi to fall asleep that night. We hope it is due to a combination of jetlag and reorienting to her bed and nighttime routine. But as Matt and I stand over her crib, as we've done every night since she was born, we can tell that she is already getting weaker and that it is hard for her to get comfortable. She lifts her head just barely enough to turn it to the other side. Back and forth she turns, slowly, until she finds her perfect spot.

Seeing the weakness in her neck reminds me that when she was born, and the midwife placed her on my chest, she immediately lifted her head up to look at Matt and me, and the nurses and midwives couldn't believe her strength. In fact, they each told us, they had never seen a newborn lift her head the way Havi did. Now, seventeen months later, she can barely lift her neck to get in a comfortable sleeping position. Back and forth, back and forth she turns. *Hush*, we whisper, and rub her back and write words on her belly with our fingers—something my parents used to do when I was young. From now on, whenever she has a hard time falling asleep, it becomes an excuse for me to write "I love you" to her, over and over again.

Our West Coast hiatus fades quickly into memory. Everything is moving too fast. Blyth sends us a perfectly timed note: "You will work to hold in balance 'Everyday life as normal AND the this-is-not-OK-or-normal.' And you will find pockets of beauty peeking out every day." I'd learn that

finding pockets of beauty, amidst the tragedies of life, might be the ultimate gift.

* * *

Back in Boston, we immediately have to attend several doctors' appointments—all bringing cruel reminders of our Tay-Sachs reality. Our
Havimoon allowed us to slip out of reality through a fold in time; we had
stolen a few weeks where real life couldn't find us, but now Tay-Sachs
resurfaces with its crushing powers.

Plus, it is February in Boston—another month of bleak, gray skies;
brown, slushy roads, after seemingly endless blizzards; and trees still
standing leafless, shivering in the bitter cold. Sunny days are nowhere
close by.

One of our appointments is with the obstetrics department, back at
the Brigham and Women's Hospital, for my twenty-week ultrasound to
check on Havi's little sister. Matt and I sit in the waiting room holding
hands. We don't speak. I notice several other couples, young and naïve,
cuddling and giggling. I remember us that way.

Tay-Sachs has changed everything for us, so this ultrasound appointment evokes a tumult of emotions for me. Even as I anticipate my second daughter with hope and excitement, I also have the deep anguish
of knowing that whomever this beautiful new baby is going to be, she'll
only physically share space with her older sister for a number of months.
I can't help but worry, too, that maybe the testing would be unreliable
again, and that this baby will have Tay-Sachs.

"Myra Sack?"

"Yep, here."

"Do you want to tell the tech about Havi? Just so she is as sensitive
as possible?"

"No. Let's play pretend in there." I say to Matt.

The effort to hold my full spectrum of emotions in check was exhausting. I really did not want to share anything I felt with the doctors today.

The ultrasound is a blur but it goes perfectly. Matt holds my hand
throughout the scan and seems to be listening more attentively than I can
to what the radiologist says about the baby appearing healthy and growing

and me being on track for a healthy pregnancy. But there is really no time to celebrate this miracle because the next thing we have to do is hurry off to meet Tia and Havi across the street, at Boston Children's Hospital for our first meeting with the pediatric palliative care team. Moments after seeing an image on a screen that shows us a healthy, growing fetus, we move to discuss our daughter's end-of-life plan. In the course of these two hours, we experience life's arc, from beginning to end.

The pediatric palliative care meeting takes place in a small, private conference room. The team of four providers speaks with a sense of kindness and calm, each member introducing themselves, describing how and why they have entered the field of pediatric palliative care, and, of course, commenting on Havi's beauty—in particular, they note her luminous eyes. "They're magnetic, almost mystical," one says. Their role will be to help us manage caring for Havi in our home, according to our values and our care goals, they say, and we can call on them for help navigating resources or to adjust medications to new baselines as Havi's disease progresses. This all makes sense to us. We do not want Havi in the hospital. We want her at home. Most importantly, we know she wants to be at home, and the least we can do is grant her that.

Then it is our turn to talk. "Tell us about Havi," the social worker prompts, inviting us to share.

I try to start, but only get as far as "She is incredible," before bursting into tears and needing Matt to take over.

Matt then bravely shares all about our girl, how she had been so strong, so capable, so curious, so full of life only a few months ago. He finishes by telling the team, "She's everything—the brightest light in our world."

We leave the meeting feeling both gratitude for a team of providers who now know Havi and will support the way we plan to live with her, and utter dejection. There is no medical intervention that enhances Havi's life. There is no hope.

We drive home in silence. Havi falls asleep in her car seat, as Tia sits next to her rubbing her cheeks and humming a lullaby. When we pull into the driveway and turn the car off, Havi wakes up. We tell Tia she should head home, and that we'll take Havi for a walk. We bundle her up in the stroller and head down our street.

I peer underneath the stroller awning to see if Havi is awake. She is. "You're going to have a sister," I tell her. "Please be okay enough to meet her."

Matt keeps walking beside us quietly. "Where are you, Emmy?"

"No place good."

"It's just a lot," he says.

* * *

We settle in for the night. Matt and Havi dance. He swings her around, dips her low, and holds her above his head as he spins around, and an hour goes by in a minute. Matt is sweaty and smiley. From Springsteen to Fleetwood Mac to DJ Khalid, we play all of what has become her favorite songs. Havi hangs onto Matt's shoulder, raises her arms, and darts her head back and forth, savoring the air. For some moments, as Matt and Havi dance, life feels the way we had imagined it was going to be. Havi has endless energy that sometimes tires us out after a long day of play, and we have to force ourselves to have serious faces to let her know that it is time for bed. We try, for her sake, to treat each day as just another full one in a life with no expiration date, but our reality is inescapable. We live in a house that we never needed to baby-proof, with a brand-new basketball hoop installed outside that Havi will never use, and many of her toys piled in their unopened boxes in the corner of her closet, for they are all toys that had been meant for a beautiful baby girl who could walk and run.

CHAPTER 13

Unity of Opposites

We celebrate Havi's tenth Shabbirthday in Boston on February 21. She hits the double digits! My parents fly up from Philadelphia, and Havi spends most of the day swept up in her Grandi and Grandadder's love. The three of them disappear to play and we don't hear from them for hours. Then they emerge, each one's smile bigger than the other. Grandi says that being with Havi is "like getting a heart massage."

Before we know it, it is time for bed, and bedtimes are getting harder. Putting Havi down to sleep means that another day has come and gone, one fewer for her to be with us. Each "goodnight" feels like a dress rehearsal for our eventual goodbye, and my chest hurts every time we walk out of her room and click off the light.

Still, being at home in Boston, we settle into a routine of beautiful mornings. Havi's little sounds wake us early and Matt is usually the first up to go and scoop her out of bed.

This week, in Matt's letter to Havi, he recounts their mornings together and considers the new world we need to make—one that holds the unity of opposites, not only happy things or only sad things, but all things.

> Dear Peanut,
>
> We go in for a snuggle with Mom before heading downstairs to breakfast. You start with blueberries or kiwi fruit followed by something from the "hot buffet," as Mom likes to call it—cheesy eggs, blueberry pancakes, French toast. Last Thursday morning I sleepily screwed up the blueberry pancake recipe, forgetting several ingredients. Your pancakes were more like blueberry breakfast tortillas that quickly burned and set off the smoke alarm. Your mom came

running in, looking panicked, and you sat oh so calmly in your new cupcake beanie and smiled at all the fuss. Thanks for being patient with me. And you ate the pancakes anyway, which I appreciated.

That night, just after we turned off the bedside light and settled onto our pillows, taking deep breaths after another day come and gone, your mom whispered to me, "Do you feel like she's slipping from us?" In the quiet pause that followed, you let out the most fantastic yawlp, which made us laugh and simultaneously ejected us both out of bed and into your room. You were lying there quietly on your back, and you looked up at us with your biggest eyes and the slightest smile. We get it, you're very much still here with us, Peanut.

As we stood in your room, your mom reached over to me and gently grabbed my hand. She guided it quietly to her belly and said, "Here, feel right here." In the quiet darkness, your little sister kicked up against my palm, ever so gently. I remembered so clearly the first time I felt you kick. Your mom and I were sitting on the sagging brown couch in our apartment on Centre Street. It was early evening, in that time between the workday and dinner. When your mom put my hand on her stomach, I couldn't believe it. I got teary eyed, which your mom thought was cute, and we talked about what bringing you into the world was going to mean.

I don't know how we're going to be able to hold both your sister's arrival and your leaving us. These two things are so impossibly opposing, just like the familiar roads around our house that now feel so unfamiliar. This week I started reading Dr. Joanne Cacciatore's book, *Bearing the Unbearable*, and there was something Dr. Jo said that I liked. Your mom's friend sent us Dr. Jo's book after your diagnosis, and we are making it required reading for our whole family. This particular passage was about the unity of opposites: Being happy does not mean we do not feel pain or grief or sadness—successively or, as happens more often, simultaneously. Sorrow and contentment, grief and beauty, longing and surrender coexist in the realm of sameness. This is called the unity of opposites, and it liberates us from a myopic, dualistic view of our emotions as either/or.

Our new world is a both/and world, Peanut.

I love you.

Dad

*   *   *

At the end of February, it is time to vote in the primary elections. At lunchtime, I drive to our polling station at the local elementary school, park the car, and look around at the scene before me. The playground is filled with kids running around at recess. I take a deep breath and feel my inhalation get caught somewhere between my breastbone and throat. I get out of the car and walk as quickly as possible, head down, toward the building. Although I am not looking at the kids anymore, I can still hear their happy shouts. It hurts just the same.

The truth is that leaving home for even a short period of time is beginning to require a lot of energy and courage. Today, I convince myself that voting is important, and that perhaps undertaking an act of expansion, rather than one of contraction, will do me some good. The trouble with expansion, though, is that you can't control what's out there in the expanding world.

As I make it to the front steps of the school, I am stopped by a mother collecting signatures about a local issue. She is blocking the door so I have no choice but to engage in small talk. She asks about Havi—well, not by name, but she wants to know where I live and whether we have kids she may have seen out on the street. I swallow hard and give her a very partial answer, "We have an eighteen-month-old daughter."

Suddenly, I feel angry for Havi. Before the other mom has a chance to unleash on me the inevitable string of classic questions about toddlers—"Is she walking?" "How many words does she have?" "Is she in preschool?"—I smile and wish her well and squeeze around her to enter the building and make my way to the voting booth.

After casting my vote, I race back down the steps, avoiding any further conversation with the woman collecting signatures, anxious to make it home, desperate to have Havi back in my arms. Once I am there again, holding her, my breathing becomes a little more natural, a little less forced.

Sometimes, as I hold Havi, I watch the gentle rise and fall of her abdomen, and I try to match her effortless breathing because it makes me feel closer to her.

In bed, I tell Matt that I am scared of losing the ability to hold her so close, to smell her skin, feel her hair, and hear her littlest sounds that we can only hear when we are right up close to her.

Matt says, "Keep holding onto her as much and as often as you can."

"Yeah. You're right," I reply. But I am unsatisfied.

* * *

As February draws to a close, Matt and I return to our respective jobs. Our incredible employers had granted us the flexibility to be in California on the Havimoon, and they are continuing to give us latitude to work remotely. It is the greatest gift we can imagine, for which we know we will forever be grateful. But it is not easy to be back in the working world, and neither Matt nor I feel particularly good about it.

Often it seems as if we are simply going through the motions at work, and that too feels bad to both of us. Matt and I both care about our work and our professional communities. Matt pursued immuno-oncology research in an MD/PhD program at Stanford which he'd planned to tackle during his career. He is now a doctor and a scientist, and an incredibly effective leader, working within a network of professional mentors who believe in his potential. I love the way he talks about science and medicine and how deeply passionate he is about changing the course of cancer in our lifetime. He loves his work, and it suits him. But now he is lost. I've never seen this vacancy in him. And it scares me.

I feel similarly. Work has been a vocation for me. I had long imagined one day leading a nonprofit organization that closed the opportunity gap for young people in the United States. I believe this could be done through the power of sports and education in combination with enduring, intensive, and meaningful adult and peer relationships. I believe that if we leverage the same kind of devotion and resources to young people in all communities as we do for families living in affluent neighborhoods, we can change the face of this country. I had long wanted to be part of that—and to be a leader of this change in Boston. But now, all I want is for my family to be okay. All I want are as many full days as possible with my daughter. This inward focus is new for me. I feel small and selfish, but it is the only way I can get through the day.

So Matt and I do the best we can, given the circumstances. We work as much as we are able without sacrificing too much time with Havi, and we feel okay knowing that for the few hours when we do have to leave the house, she is with Tia.

During this time of transition, Leah arrives from Dallas. Her timing is divine. Sleep has become increasingly challenging for Havi, and on the first night of what becomes a sleep-strike, Leah decides to creep into Havi's room and join her, literally. Matt walks in to find Leah curled up on the floor with a blanket and a pillow right next to Havi's crib. The two of them peek up at him from their respective beds and smile. Busted!

The next night, just as we are getting Havi ready for bed, Leah comes back into her room dragging a beanbag chair, two blankets, and a pillow. Sleepover night two is about to begin. I don't think either one of them does much sleeping though, as Havi spends most of the night curled up in her Aunt Leah's arms. I fall asleep down the hall imagining the two of them giggling and hatching secret plans that Matt and I will never be privy to.

Since we are in a losing race against time, we cherish everything to do with Havi: every smile, cuddle, meal, every blink and flutter of her beautiful eyelashes. So, when one of her eyelashes falls to rest on her cheek or her nose, we race to pick it up and make a wish for her, blowing the eyelash and the wish out into the universe. According to tradition, we can't tell anyone else those wishes.

CHAPTER 14

Restless

It's still very much winter in Boston. Matt has been growing restless. In a pressured exchange that feels like a cry for help, he convinces/begs me to make one more trip back West. He says he wants to see family and treat Havi to more experiences at the ocean and in the hot tub, and to savor a few final sunsets together. But I know deep down there is something escapist in his travel urges too. We fly back to San Francisco on March 7, 2020.

Our plan is to spend two weeks away: one in California with Jacob and Erin and Havi's Grandma and Grandpa, and another in Dallas visiting Leah and Mike. Then we will head back to Boston for good. For the final part of Havi's life arc. At this point, there are murmurings of Covid-19, but nobody has any real understanding of the virus or appreciation of what lies ahead once the pandemic spreads around the world.

It is drizzling in Boston on the morning we leave and the weather isn't much better when we touch down in San Francisco. In both airports, we see a handful of people wearing masks, which we assume is out of an abundance of caution, but the vast majority of people, including us, are unmasked and look unconcerned. There are currently nineteen US deaths due to Covid-19.

Jacob and Erin surprise us at the airport, holding a sign bearing Havi's name. My eyes well up with tears when I see them, and Havi smiles and settles easily into Erin's arms. As we head to Matt's parents' house, the gray clouds give way to a big blue sky. It is cool outside when we arrive, but the sunlight is strong and we stand out on the patio for a few minutes to take big gulps of the northern California air that smells like oak and eucalyptus. I feel Havi's shoulders relax and she leans into me. It is naptime. She settles right into the new time zone.

On the day of Havi's thirteenth Shabbirthday, we go to Half Moon Bay for lunch with Grandma and sit at a little table overlooking the waves, happy to be at the ocean again with Havi. After she finishes her lunch of sourdough bread and cheesy eggs, her eyes grow heavy in the warm sun, so I slide her into the stroller, where she sleeps for over an hour with the sound of the waves in her ears. When she awakes again, as we stand looking out to sea, Grandma Marilyn catches sight of the puff of a whale's waterspout about a hundred yards out. Then a big, blue, arching back appears—a humpback whale is bobbing and playing just beyond the surf. We watch for a while and as we are about to turn and leave, the massive creature raises itself straight up out of the water, its head pointing toward the sky, and hangs there for a beautiful second, looking at us. "Look, Havi," I say, "that whale is saying hello to you!"

Every Shabbirthday is sacred, but this one seems to carry an extra special dose of holiness. It is the thirteenth one, so we honor it as if it were Havi's Bat Mitzvah.

Dear Peanut,

You are getting older, and we're watching you closely, trying to capture every little change. The Bat Mitzvah is a big day in the life a young Jewish person. I was a little peanut, just like you, when I made my Bar Mitzvah and I could barely see over the podium at the synagogue. Like most kids, I was more excited about the party that followed than I was appreciating the intensity of the transition—going from a boy to a man in g-d's eyes. This past week I thought a lot about what that day must have meant for my parents, your grandparents. And I tried to imagine what your Bat Mitzvah would have been like for us: A big stack of blueberry pancakes before we all got dressed up and headed to the synagogue; you walking up to stand in front of the congregation, so poised and confident; you leading us through the service with laughter and grace and then heaving a big sigh of relief when your Torah portion was done.

I've thought about your Bat Mitvah a lot this week. I don't know what to call these visits I pay to the beautiful future that I still imagine for you—I told your mom that maybe they are "fore-memories." She said, "I think they're called dreams." So, yes, I've been visiting you in my dreams and it's been crushingly painful and yet so beautiful. Someday maybe we'll meet each other there.

This week, your Grandi and Grandadders asked their local Rabbi, Shelly Barnathan, to share a few words on this week's Torah portion. She wrote us a beautiful note and I've copied some of it here for you:

Havi, your Bat Mitzvah Torah portion is Ki Tisa, which means, "when you lift, or when you count." The *parashah* is about the equal portion—the half-shekel that each Israelite was asked to contribute in the wilderness to create the Mishkan, the holy traveling sanctuary. Creating the Mishkan was a community effort, holy work that was done together.

Havi, the Mishkan held holiness, and in order to create holiness, each person was asked to contribute both an equal share and also something special and unique from his, her, or their own heart. And when each person contributed in both of these ways, then, like the title of the Torah portion, "Ki Tisa," says, each person's soul was "lifted up" and each person "counted"—one just as much as the other.

Havi, you are a Mishkan, a source of holiness. You radiate light with your smile and your giggles. You receive and offer love, and you lift up others with the purity of your Neshama, your pure, sweet soul. You count in this world, dear Havi Lev!

So with that blessing, Peanut, Shabbat was upon us. Grandma and Grandpa made an incredible dinner with all of Matt's favorite foods and your Aunt Maggie arrived from Colorado and baked two delicious challahs for you to gobble up. One was chocolate chip! (Mom and I did some advance sampling of that loaf. We hope you understand.) Your Aunt Erin and Uncle Jacob came and our good friend Brendan was there too. We read Rabbi Shelly's words, gazed at the incredible Tree of Life photo collage that Jacob and Erin created, and stuffed ourselves with Maggie's challah. We celebrated you as our Bat Mitzvah girl and held you extra tight as we danced the night away.

Love you, Peanut.

Dad

CHAPTER 15

Covid by the Bay

On March 11, 2020 the World Health Organization declares Covid-19 a pandemic. On March 19, 2020, California issues a statewide stay-at-home order. The incidence of Covid-19 is rising here. We have to cancel our trip to Dallas, where we had planned to visit Leah and Mike before returning to Boston.

Instead, we decide to escape the growing madness of San Francisco, where the lockdown is making it difficult and scary to go outside, and travel farther north to Tomales Bay, intending to spend only a few days there. Ordinarily, we don't travel around in the simple pursuit of beautiful places, but caring for a dying child changes the way you think about the next right thing. Now, we'll shelter-in-place there until it is safe to head back to Boston. We can't take any risks with Havi, a severe infection could be devastating, so we live day-to-day. Jacob and Erin, who are living in San Francisco, will join us there. The move makes sense because all of our jobs have suddenly gone fully remote.

After loading up on groceries and essentials we drive two hours to a beautiful little cottage perched on the edge of the bay. The cottage is unassuming from the front, with brown shingles and a tall, heavy fence that blocks it from US-1 highway, which is normally busy, but because of Covid-19, has no traffic. I am immediately charmed by the front doorknob shaped like a ship's wheel. Inside, there are big windows along the back of the house, offering a breathtaking view of Tomales Bay. We can see Point Reyes National Seashore in the distance. The cottage is only about a thousand square feet, but our outdoor playground is endless.

We settle into a new, quiet, routine as the entire world spins into overdrive, overwhelmed by sickness and struggles. I feel completely ill-equipped to grasp the severity of Covid. The gravity of the situation is ever evolving and beyond my comprehension, but it certainly offers us a reminder of how connected we all are to one another and the incredible power and responsibility that comes along with that interconnectedness. Maybe most dramatically, the pandemic reveals that true compassion calls for an ability to care about people you've never met and may never meet. Never in my lifetime has it been so obvious that another person's actions or inactions could have such a profound ripple effect on the health or well-being of a complete stranger. Covid-19 feels like it could be controlled, or perhaps contained, if everyone stares into the eyes of someone they are about to lose and promises that they'll follow whatever necessary guidelines to prevent that. I can see that kind of compassion in Havi's eyes, and hope it is contagious. Her brightness and love make Matt and me want to be better to each other and to the world. Every day she is teaching us to be more patient, loving, observant, and present. I wish I didn't have to learn these lessons this way.

Out on the bay the air is clean and crisp and the colors are vibrant, with beautiful birds fanning their wings through the sky. At our cottage Havi likes to sit in front of the big window that looks out over the water, eating her meals above the waves with the sun shining on her back. Even more than usual, I find her very being mesmerizing. The bay is quiet, peaceful, soft, and majestic—it feels a lot like Havi. And whenever I am brave and vulnerable enough, I stand with her and let the softness of the air, the fullness of the sun, and the gentle motion of the waves work their healing powers on me. But it is hard and painful to sit in all that calmness.

Every day we take Havi some place beautiful. Our first stop is the Bear Valley Train in Point Reyes National Park. Initially, Havi makes a pretty strong case against ever going in her stroller again. She cries so hard that she convinces some passersby that Matt and I are highly inept caretakers as we move her back and forth between the stroller, the carrier Matt is wearing, and my arms. Still, she is unhappy. But finally, in an instant it seems, she falls fast asleep in the carrier against Matt's chest and lies snuggled up against him for over an hour as we walk along the dirt trail lined with cypress, oak, and eucalyptus trees. After today, we decide, we will leave the stroller in the car.

We show Havi all around Point Reyes, bobbing and weaving on paths that range through woods and fields and along beaches, walking beside cows and sheep that graze on hills you couldn't possibly paint a more beautiful green. Each time we tuck Havi into the carrier, she holds her head against Matt's chest and peers out at the beautiful world. Any chance he has, Matt kisses her hands and her forehead, sometimes so hard that he says his nose tingles. He tells me he wants to imprint his every sense with her so he'll never forget.

One afternoon, as we drive back to our cottage after another beautiful hike, Havi starts to fuss and squirm and moments later, she throws up. Matt, who is sitting in the backseat next to her as I drive, catches a lot of the vomit in his hand and on his lap. Food goes the wrong way sometimes for everyone, but the stakes are higher for Havi, and Matt and I are both shaken up. We know she is at a greater risk of developing aspiration pneumonia, which occurs when food, saliva, liquid, or vomit is breathed into the lungs instead of being swallowed down the esophagus and into the stomach.

Fortunately, Matt breaks our uneasy silence with a joke: "Maybe it is your driving, My."

I laugh and feel like my old self for a moment. But in Matt's lap lay a lot of Havi's lunch, in big, unchewed chunks. Despite the soft foods we've been giving her and the small bites we've seen her taking, it is clear that Havi has been swallowing everything whole and smiling through it. We know that at some point we'll have to transition to blended meals for her, but we have pushed that thought away. Just five or six months earlier she had been feeding herself blueberries in the morning. Now we realize we need to buy a cheap blender from the general store near the bay.

Not yet, Matt and I say to each other with our eyes. *Please, not yet.* We are scared as hell to lose her.

* * *

Meanwhile, Covid-19 rages. The death toll climbs above 200,000 deaths and a vaccine seems out of reach, so Matt and Jacob and Erin and I hunker down for a while longer in our little cottage on Tomales Bay. The pandemic has made it impossible for people to travel, so we decide to take full advantage of the situation. By then we have been on the bay for a whole month, and every week, as we extend the rental yet again, the price steadily drops. Occasionally Jacob and Erin head back to San Francisco to pick up more clothes and supplies from their apartment, but Matt and I stay put, and we all agree that it is safer to be out of the city and on the bay.

Plus, Havi loves it out here by the water, which makes it easy to continue adjusting our rhythm to the shifting tides. Sometimes I wish we could stay here forever. Whenever we step out into the salty wind that comes whooshing over the bay from the Pacific, she closes her eyes and opens her mouth wide to taste it. The sounds of the natural world are clearer on the bay and it does well to drown out some of the chaos that has engulfed the rest of our planet.

Every morning, Havi gets excited about watching the resident otter slip and spin through the water just off the dock. We name him, "Mr. Otter," and he becomes a friend. We count on him to jump up to say hello every morning. It feels like Havi's existence matters to Mr. Otter. We love that.

But the morning after Havi vomits on Matt, she wakes up with a high fever, and we feel like we are inching closer and closer to the edge of a cliff. After twenty-four hours her fever breaks. We make an appointment for a virtual visit with Amanda Hull, Havi's speech-language pathologist/feeding specialist, who has already given us some helpful guidance on what to feed Havi and how to prepare it.

Amanda reinforces what we already know: Havi's meals will have to be soft and mashed, and we need to start thickening her fluids to make them easier to swallow. Even though Havi is eating better again, and has even devoured several sweet potatoes, it is clear that we are in a new phase.

That truth really comes home to us one Friday morning when Matt wakes up early to make Havi her Shabbirthday pancakes. He lines up all of the ingredients on the counter and whips up the batter. Soon, three perfect Havi-sized pancakes are sizzling in the pan. But as Matt reaches for the blueberries to add them to the cooking pancakes, he thinks again, and stops short. Whole blueberries are out. In a moment of anguish and rage, Matt throws them all into the garbage. Then he gathers himself and pours a big scoop of warm blueberry jam onto Havi's plate instead and dips every little bite of mashed-up pancake into it before feeding it to her.

By now the national parks are closed, with their parking lot entrances blocked and caution tape strung across the beginnings of trails, but we still bring Havi out for hikes. We make these beautiful places ours forever—they are now home to our memories of the ephemeral and enchanting time we spend with Havi in this bubble, surrounded by the oak- and eucalyptus-covered coastal mountains and sea mist in the mornings, witnessing stunning sunsets marking the end of every day.

One day we all drive out to the end of the Point Reyes wilderness and park on the edge of a large meadow dotted with cows. I tuck Havi into the chest carrier and Matt and Erin and Jacob and I hike out with her along the edge of a lagoon rimmed with wildflowers, then over the sand dunes, past a couple of otters rolling around in the rushes by the shoreline, right out to the tip of the land stretching out into the ocean. At some point, her breathing gets heavy and slows and her head weighs heavily against my chest. The ocean has put her to sleep. We walk alongside the waves and watch a flock of little white birds darting in and out of the water, zigzagging in perfect synchrony. Erin carves Havi's initials, HLG, into the sand and we pose for pictures, standing around it with the Pacific at our backs.

Then we decide to turn for home, and as we start to leave the beach, a big wave crashes behind us. We all turn to see Havi's initials in the sand being covered in foam and then wash away as the wave recedes.

* * *

April 11, 2020

Sweets,

I've been staring at your mom a lot this week too. She, quite all of sudden, is looking very pregnant with your baby sister. So maybe it's that, or maybe it's the deepening tan of a few weeks in the California sun, or maybe it's the couple of good nights of sleep that you've given us this week, but regardless, your mom has been looking particularly beautiful this week. You fit so perfectly together—you tucked into her arms, your cheeks gently touching hers, and your light golden curls weaving in between the cascading strands of her smooth brown hair. All of the minutes in every day will never be long enough for me to watch the two of you.

So when your Mom came in through the front gate with

tears streaming down her cheeks, and her knees and hands scraped and bleeding and covered in dirt, I panicked. Your mom—at twenty-seven weeks pregnant, mind you—was putting down 7:20 miles running the steep descent of the Marshall-Petaluma road when she fell and sprained her ankle—and clearly did all kinds of contortions not to land on her pregnant belly. So we cleaned Mom up. She was pretty shaken and so worried about your baby sister. She wouldn't move from the chair in the kitchen, sipping water, until she felt kicks again. And then we all sat together, Jacob and Erin and you and me, as the sun set over the water, and we took turns putting our hands on Mom's belly to feel your baby sister moving around. I'm not sure whether you felt the kicks or not, but I think you know our little family is growing. And maybe that's why you've been so giggly this week.

Love you, Peanut.

Dad

CHAPTER 16

Tension and Laughter

Inevitably, mealtime arrives and we spend a wonderfully long time watching Havi delight in her food and the kisses we give her between bites. One day, as we make our way through a meal, Havi's shirt slips off her shoulder and I am struck by how much her little body has already withered. She is only nineteen months old. There will be no growth curves or developmental milestones for Havi.

The reality of the brutally short time we have left together is so painful that it sometimes incapacitates me, and I spend the day in bed with a book. Our family's future has been shattered into a thousand pieces that lie strewn about and it seems impossible to even begin to pick them up, let alone figure out how to rebuild our life. And so a battle rages on in my head and in my heart, as love and life struggle against grief and death, jerking me back and forth, or even worse, leaving me quivering in the middle of all those terrible feelings.

At the end of every day comes nighttime. Our routine begins with saying a proper goodnight to Tomales Bay. I carry Havi out to the dock and say goodnight to all her new friends.

Say goodnight to the Bay.

Say goodnight to the oysters and the swallows that live beneath us; to the grey heron and the white heron and the pelican and the seagulls and don't forget the common loon!

Say goodnight to Mr. Otter and to the slippery seal. And to hog island and piglet island and the flying pigs.

Say goodnight to the water and the wind and the land and the sunset.

And they all say, "Goodnight Sweet Hav. We love you so much, sleep so well, and we'll see you in the morning."

Then I hand her to Matt who gives her an extra squeeze. Havi's golden hair blows in the wind and her eyes get heavy.

We go back inside, find Jacob and Erin for goodnight kisses, and then Matt carries her into her bedroom, a narrow room with a set of bunkbeds and a crib and rocker. Instead of a bedtime bottle of warm milk, Havi drinks a carefully mixed, perfectly viscous milkshake. Matt places her on my lap, and covers her pajamas with several towels of different shapes, sizes, and wicking power to absorb the pools of liquid that otherwise end up soaking her. Then Matt and I take turns burping and rocking her and together we tuck her into the small toddler rocker that Grandma gave to us. We try to ignore the significance of abandoning her crib, focusing instead on making her comfy cozy. In the crib, she wakes up every thirty minutes struggling to breathe. The upright position of the rocker is safer and for now we all feel better. Sort of.

Eventually, with us watching over her, she falls asleep. We gently close her door and collapse into each other's arms, meeting somewhere between exhaustion, heartbreak, fear, and infinite love. After a few good cries, I look over at Matt: "Ice cream?"

"Yes, always," I say. Thank goodness for ice cream. And for poetry, which has become a new devotion for us after a friend recommended it as a powerful container for grief. Life on the bay is just what we need it to be.

Meanwhile, in addition to spending time with Havi, our dailyness includes work. And work has morphed into a series of Zoom calls for all of us. Jacob, Erin, Matt, and I rotate through various positions in our little cottage: at the kitchen table, at the picnic table outside, in our respective bedrooms—or my favorite, the walking call, taken in laps around the house. We never compromise Havi's eating schedule or comfort. Sometimes she is curled up on one of our laps while we finish a Zoom call or write an email; other times, we pass her back and forth as we navigate overlapping calls. In between spates of work, we find brief but big moments to dance and smile with her. *Brief but big:* We only have that.

As the days on the bay tick by, we are fortunate for visits from Grandma and Grandpa, who drive up the coast from Matt's childhood home and enter our bubble for afternoon walks along the water. But our existence with Havi becomes more and more isolated from the everyday outside world. We are creating our own reality; one that is hyper-present and hyper-aware. Hugging, holding, kissing Havi feels imperative on a cellular level and I am immersed in her. I've never lived this way and it's beautiful.

In our tiny cottage perched on the edge of Tomales Bay, in the middle of a pandemic, it's easy for Havi, Matt, Jacob, Erin, and me to exist in this bubble. But at some point, I realize that I'm starting to feel irritated with Jacob. He's my brother, after all, so annoyance is part of the rhythm of our existence, but my ability to manage these feelings now is lower than it has ever been. Jacob is firmly in our bubble but he has a foot in the everyday world too. His calendar is full and he's on the phone a lot. I can see the intensity of ambition and accomplishment pulse around him whenever our paths cross during the day. One evening I overhear him and Erin talking about a promotion that Jacob has been gunning for and now has indications that he's likely to receive. My simmering annoyance is growing to a boil. I couldn't care less. And I'm genuinely confused as to how he can work this much or care about work this much when we're living the lesson that it truly doesn't matter.

I start by being passive aggressive, not making eye contact, cutting conversations short, making unprompted jabs about how stupid his job is, and then finally I snap. "Fuck you, Jacob! Your meetings don't matter and they're dumb," I yell, marching across the kitchen into our bedroom. There isn't much of a place to hide in our 1,000 square foot cottage.

"Okay, Fra," Jacob says, using the childhood nickname coined from the way he once described my running endurance relative to his: "She just fra-la-las along," he said. And "Fra" stuck. I can see him through the gap between the door and the frame standing, looking down at his feet. He's an amazing big brother and I know he's trying to figure out what to say to make it better. I should go back out and talk with him but I don't. The next day we agree to meet out on the deck after Havi is asleep to talk.

He starts to apologize, and I cut him off. "Sometimes I just feel like you don't get it, Jacob. And then I get angry with you and then I feel bad because I know you're trying and doing everything. I just don't understand how you can care about these things now."

I want to be able to get excited for him, to celebrate his professional accomplishments and admire his ambition. But I can't; it infuriates me. And I am defensive. I need to protect Havi and our little bubble from everything and anything that can distract from our focus on her. Her moments on this earth with me number in months, days, minutes, and I want every single one of them to be filled with the fullest love. So, in that moment, looking across at the brother who will do anything for me, who has done everything for me, I make the decision that the only people who can enter Havi's orbit are those people who are fully in. From then on, we are living in a pure no-bullshit zone.

*　*　*

April 18, 2020

Dear Beauty,

We had another first this week, sweet girl.

Dad wanted a haircut. Excitedly, he asked me if I'd be his barber. I was honored. We put you down for bed, and Dad set up shop. He brought a chair outside on the deck, covered it with a towel, and meticulously laid out the shiny new at-home haircutting tool kit that was miraculously available at our tiny little local pharmacy: blades, guards, a comb, and scissors. We talked through the various instruments, and he described the difference between a quarter-inch guard, one-inch guard, and everything in between. We stood in front of the mirror and Dad showed me how the barber at home uses the comb and scissors together, and the steady, calculated approach to a great haircut. You can imagine, Dad didn't miss a single instruction.

He sat down in the chair. I held the half-inch guard in my hand, my heart racing in anticipation, and my deadpan expression masking all anxiety or insecurity. Now wasn't the time for self-doubt; I had to be confident. And then, we were in it, hair started to fall on Dad's shoulders and sides needed to be evened out. I was Dad's barber! And things were looking pretty good, until...well, midway through this gorgeous

78

haircut, you woke up and I went in to soothe you. You were cheering us on! When I returned, Dad had decided to clean the razor (not a surprise) and had taken the guard off in the process. He mentioned this to me as he sat back down but I wasn't listening carefully enough. So, I swiftly grabbed what I thought was the half-inch guard and in one fell swoop, cleaned up his left side. Only, the razor didn't have a guard on it! So the left side of Dad's head was shaved to skin in one fluid stroke. He now looks like an edgy punk pseudo skater boy. No offense to skater boys, it's a different kind of look for your dad.

We laughed so hard we both went to bed with stomach aches. The good kinds. As we laughed together with our heads on our pillows, I said I couldn't remember the last time we had laughed that hard—the kind of laughter where you have to cross your legs and clench and hope that you don't pee. It was a good reminder for us that we, too, still have laughter in us. Maybe you passed your giggles our way this week. You probably knew we needed them. So, thank you.

And thanks to your dad, for being the most remarkably loving, patient, and thoughtful person in the world. I am reminded in so many moments of every day, and in particular, every morning when he leaves a cup of perfectly modified London Fog tea (English Breakfast, not Early Grey) awaiting me on my bedside table. And trust me, Hav, you'd be so amazed by all the ways he takes care of you every day. It's his greatest joy. My former students called him Superman, and they were so right.

PART
III

"Life is about a joyful participation
in a world of sorrows."

PICO IYER

CHAPTER 17

Setsunai

It is the end of April, more than a month and a half after we first arrived in California for what was meant to be a week-long stay. We are burning through our savings and despite the support of Erin and Jacob are struggling to manage caring for Havi with daily work schedules that are now filled with zoom calls. So, begrudgingly, we book flights to return home to Boston and let the Airbnb host know that we will be checking out of our little haven on the bay.

Within hours, a United Airlines alert shows up on Matt's cell phone that our flight back to Boston has been cancelled due to Covid. We are relieved and take this as a very clear sign that it is not yet time to leave the bay. So we call the Airbnb host back again and hope that he'll agree to a rate that makes staying feasible. Matt drives back out to the little grocery store, Palace Market, in Point Reyes Station to stock up on peanut butter, applesauce, and the single roll of toilet paper each customer is allotted per day.

That afternoon, as the sun starts to move toward the horizon, I take Havi back out to the deck and we resume our search for Mr. Otter. Staying on the bay means more mornings of waking up to the sound of the water lapping against the rocks and more evenings watching the sun sparkle on the bay and then drop behind the hills of Point Reyes to the ocean beyond. It means more of Havi's giggles over long meals with Jacob and Erin. So we are still able to maintain our little, magical time bubble out here on the bay. We relish every day. It's true, it feels like Havi laughs more here than she has in her entire life, like we all laugh here more than we have in our entire lives. Nature nourishes and regenerates.

A few days later, after the excitement and relief of having to extend our stay has worn off, I walk out onto the deck one afternoon and find that Matt's face is dark and serious. "What's going on, babe?" I ask.

Matt doesn't want to leave. And not just in a few weeks. He doesn't want to leave ever. He doesn't want to go back to Boston. I'll learn later that Boston holds deep pain, guilt, and an existential trauma around his identity as a physician. But for now, I'm only sensing that he's hesitant to give up our beautiful view, the warm California sun, and a place Havi seems to be at peace.

We have a baby on the way and I feel strongly pulled to deliver her with Dr. Grant. She is one of the only people in the medical system who feels safe to me. I also know that when we bring this new baby home, to the same house we brought Havi home to, that Tia will be there to scoop her up immediately and welcome our new person with the biggest love. There's Charlie and Blyth, who with every call and email are feeling more and more like a lifeline. And my parents reassure us that they'll be wherever we need them.

We do spend a handful of nights discussing options for selling our house in Boston and staying out in California. Matt even calls a local real estate agent and I find myself one afternoon walking through a house in some beautiful woods not too far from our cottage on the bay. Could we stay? Could we resettle our lives out here? Is this where Havi wants us to be? What should we do, sweet girl?

We FaceTime with Charlie and Blyth and share our fears about leaving the bay. Life is good to Havi here. "What happens if we get back to Boston and she stops smiling?" Matt says with fear in his voice.

Charlie pauses, then says, "A little while before Cameron died, I was with her in her room. I had turned away from her and was putting something away in her dresser when I was overcome by this sensation that she was smiling at me. I said out loud, 'I see you smiling at me beautiful girl.' Of course, it had been many months since she had smiled but every sense in my body was telling me that she had."

I see his eyes getting moist with emotion. I know we're in a unique space with Charlie and Blyth because of how similar our experiences are, separated by twenty years. But it is clear that they are on this journey with us, walking alongside and helping us to hold the weight of Havi's diagnosis. *With us.* They are more than just a sounding board or a source of advice. They are more than a couple with a shared experience of the illness and death of a child. They are part of our little peloton surrounding Havi.

A few weeks later, as we watch the sunset over the bay, we agree that we will return to Boston.

* * *

As we prepare for our eventual, impending return, which coincides with the weekend of Havi's twentieth Shabbirthday, on May 2, Matt discovers the Japanese word *Setsunai,* which means the ability to carry joy and sorrow at once, in Nina Li Coomes' column, "Mistranslate." Coomes' explanation of the word captures our feelings about going home:

> *Setsunai* carries an implication of something once bright, now faded. It is the painful twinge at the edge of a memory of someone you have loved—say, the memory of a Saturday spent together running errands, or a brilliant peel of a smile tossed at you over the lunch table—all the while knowing that person is no longer with you. It is the sting of time passing. It is the joy afloat in the knowledge that everything is temporary. Perhaps, then, the cutting implicit in *Setsunai* is the way the passage of time eventually draws a thin line of blood, of pain, across even the roundest, fullest happiness.[1]

The sting of time passing.

* * *

Jacob and Erin work their magic for Havi's twentieth Shabbirthday, her last one to be celebrated on the bay: Matt and Havi and I wake up to find a beautifully decorated kitchen table and a plate of homemade blueberry muffins, each one with "20" written in icing on top. After dinner, we break out into a mini dance party, with Havi in the middle of our circle and the four of us taking turns lifting her up into the air in pure bliss. We take

---

[1] Nina Coomes, "Setsunai: When You Need a Word to Hold both Sorrow and Joy," *Catapult* magazine, February 26, 2018, at catapult.co.

Havi outside afterwards to say goodnight to the bay for a final time, and then snuggle her off to sleep.

Whatever would come next, we'd keep our time on the bay close to us and do everything possible to create the same peace and joy wherever we are. We learn out here that life isn't about chasing extraordinary moments—it is about recognizing seemingly mundane moments as extraordinary.

For our final weekend on the bay, Jacob and Matt run the first annual "Havi Half Marathon." They chart a 13.1-mile course from Petaluma to our cottage. The first seven miles meander through cow pastures and rolling hills dotted with orange poppies. At the seven-mile mark, the road changes from flat to climb and Matt and Jacob name this stretch "Havi's Hill," which takes them all the way to mile ten. From the top of Havi's Hill, views of the world of West Marin unfold: Tomales Bay stretches to the left with the dark-green pine-covered hills that make up Point Reyes in the background; beyond that, and to the right, the Pacific stretches out as far as one can see.

Erin and I stay home during the run. When Matt and Jacob finally walk through the wooden gate, Erin and I sit in the sun and Havi is asleep in my arms. We have a celebration that Erin prepared, with a bag full of oysters, cold beers, and t-shirts from Hog Island Oyster Company, about a quarter of a mile down the road from us along the shore. I put Havi in her stroller, stand to put my arms around Matt's neck, and whisper in his ear, "Did you think about Hav?"

"The entire way," he replies, and breaks down, sobbing into my shoulder.

I hold him. I ache for him. I don't want him to know how it scares me to see him this way. Because I know he needs to cry. Havi wakes up from her nap moments later, and Matt and I gather ourselves so we can all five of us take a celebratory dip in the small cedar hot tub that Matt likes to call the 'warm pool'. As we soak in the pool, reflecting together about the run, Havi tilts her head back and sunbathes in Matt's arms.

In the middle of the following week, we all pack our suitcases to leave Tomales Bay. Erin takes Havi for a walk on the dock nearby while Matt and I pack our rental car. With the sun on her face, the wind in her hair, and Van Morrison's "Days Like This" floating from our car's speakers, Havi falls sound asleep in Erin's arms. The bay is her place.

As we drive back down Highway 1, tracking along the edge of Tomales Bay back toward San Francisco, Matt and I cry quiet tears. We spend a cozy night with Grandma and Grandpa in Matt's childhood home, and they hold Havi extra tight. We fly back to Boston in the morning. Our two months on the bay have been full of sad milestones—from when we stop giving Havi solid food to her seemingly permanent transition from sleeping in a crib to the rocker—alongside feelings of joy and Havi's many bouts of uncontrollable laughter.

"What do we do now? Back in Boston? Watch her lose everything?" Matt asks me. The questions fill me with despair but then the answer comes.

"We'll just have to say goodnight to the bay from afar and try to fill her with every bit of the peace and comfort that she has found so easily during our time out there by the sea," I say with conviction, but every ounce of me wants to curl up in my seat and make time stop.

How do you say goodbye to the things you love? You don't. You say, "See you later." So, see you later, bay.

CHAPTER 18

Mother's Day

Mother's Day morning, 2020. United Airlines flight from San Francisco to Boston.

The Covid pandemic is in full swing so we wear masks and gloves for the long flight back to the East Coast. The plane is almost empty and eerily quiet. As we rise above San Francisco Bay, I watch the outline of the Tomales Bay coastline and the ocean beyond it recede. Then the plane cabin starts to rattle with turbulence and I am shaken from my momentary daydream. I grip the armrest of my seat, close my eyes tightly, take a deep breath into my mask and tell myself: *Don't be such a wimp, My. It's a little turbulence.* When I open my eyes I peek over at Matt, holding Havi next to me and, to my surprise, Havi unleashes a smile and breaks out into laughter, looking more comfortable than ever in Matt's lap. There she is again, leading me from a place of worry to a place of humor and grace.

I take comfort in being up in the sky with Havi—it is the only place where it actually feels okay to be on Mother's Day, safely far away from other people's happiness, Hallmark cards, and nosy questions. I have never considered Mother's Day from this perspective, but now that I do, I feel extreme resentment for the holiday—for all the mothers who have lost children, for all the children who have lost their mothers, and for all the women who desperately want to become mothers but will never. We don't honor those people at all.

We touch down as a beautiful sunset lights up Boston Harbor, and I exit the plane with a mix of relief and sadness. The landing marks a dramatic end to our beautifully rich time on the West Coast and the beginning of a new and inevitably challenging chapter back home in Boston.

Tia picks us up from the airport, and although she is masked and gloved, she still holds Havi tight and smothers her with kisses. It has been several months since they have been together. "Even more beautiful, how is that possible?" Tia's warmth, devotion, and unwavering love for Havi once again lifts our spirits. As she drives us home along the familiar route, we all remark how eerie the suddenly uncongested roads are—only the pandemic can bring about a change this dramatic.

Our house looks nice and inviting as we pull into the driveway. The weather is warm, and bright green spring leaves have filled out many of the trees; in the light breeze, the trees' branches wave gently as if to say, *Welcome back.* Just opposite Havi's bedroom window, across the driveway, there is a new and very tender little cherry tree that our neighbor Liam planted for her while we were gone. He had sent us an email after planting it, telling us that despite its young state, the cherry tree is already full of blossoms.

Throughout our first week back we struggle to find a new routine: Our old ways no longer work with our new realities. But one afternoon, I see something that helps us settle in. I happen to walk into Havi's room while Tia sits with her in her white rocking chair, reading a children's book, Emily Winfield Martin's *All the Wonderful Things You'll Be.* As Tia holds up the book, I can see printed on its back cover: "This is the first time there's ever been you, so I wonder what wonderful things you will do." In a seemingly previous life, this book—which I have to admit I've always found sweet but also a bit overladen with clichéd aphorisms—has provided the perfect antidote to a hard day with Havi, but seeing it again makes my stomach clench.

Later that night, after Havi is asleep, I muster the courage to read the book again, desperate to find something that still applies to my beautiful girl. Tucked inside the front cover I find a note from Kelsey, another Dartmouth teammate who now feels like a sister. Kelsey lives in New York City and makes frequent trips to Boston to be with us and always leaves a note to Havi hidden somewhere in the house; she is Aunt Kiki to Havi and showing up comes easily and naturally to her.

"I know you'll be kind, clever and bold...and the bigger your heart, the more it will hold. The sky is the limit. I love you."

Reading Kelsey's message makes me feel a little better because it still holds true. Despite everything, Havi will become someone too. Whoever she ultimately becomes will take a different form than we could have ever imagined. It will involve a world and an imagination that transcends us, that challenges everything I ever hope for—and that tears my heart and soul apart every time I allow myself to go there. Nonetheless, Havi has a life, and it is real and rich and ours to share forever. So even though we need to do a bit of heavy editing, so to speak, her page is still somewhere to be had in Emily Winfield Martin's book.

Though Tomales Bay is now in the place of memory, we maintain our sunset routine of saying goodnight to the bay. We understand the power of daily routines, "microrituals,"[1] as a way to keep us anchored in today. So when the sun begins to set and a yawn or two sneaks out from Havi's mouth, we walk outside to say a proper goodnight to the natural world. We start with the bay and Mr. Otter and Slippery Seal, but now we have Liam's Cherry Tree too, with its ephemeral blossoms reminding us that all the beauty in this world is ever fleeting.

I go to bed anticipating my first OB appointment for our growing fetus.

---

[1] Joanne Cacciatore and Melissa Flint, "Mediating Grief: Postmortem Ritualization After Child Death," *Journal of Loss and Trauma*, 17:2 (2012), 158-172.

CHAPTER 19

Family in Boston

Havi's Twenty-third Shabbirthday: May 23, 2020

Hi Peanut,

For much of my life—or maybe all of it, really—milestones have been a dominating focal point. I remember being a little kid, maybe in third grade, standing in the outfield of Bayside Park with the wind and the fog blowing in hard off San Francisco Bay. I would look over through the chain link fence at the game being played in the neighboring field by two teams in the Babe Ruth League. The boys were big and the pitching was lively. One day that'd be me.

And so it continued. I kept my eyes up, always looking ahead to the next milestone: middle school, high school, college, medical school, residency, and so on. And when you appeared, nearly twenty-one months ago, a whole new list of milestones, which I eagerly anticipated, appeared in my life. That is, until they were delayed, or became different. And then the worst thing happened: the milestones all slipped away. Suddenly I knew there would be no milestones for you. For a moment, it had seemed like your mom and I had everything, and our world was one of progress forward, but then slowly, insidiously, everything had dissolved until the moment came when your mom and I looked at each other and realized something was not right. And since that day, we've been walking steadily backwards through and past the milestones that you had crossed before. It's tragically disorienting.

This week we abandoned your spoon and switched to feeding you with the sippy cup with the straw. Not so long ago you could use a toddler spoon, holding it in your hand and scooping food into your own mouth. But that spoon has sat in the drawer for months now, giving way to smaller spoons and smaller bites. We used to sit for hours with you, making our way through a finely mashed sweet potato; we've always cherished mealtime because you seemed to get so much joy from it. But this week we put away your last spoon and now everything gets puréed in the blender to be smooth and just thick enough for you to slurp from the sippy cup without choking.

There is a photo in our kitchen, which we hung up after we got back from our Havimoon, showing us all sitting at our daily breakfast table in Del Mar. Your hand is resting on top of a small bowl full of fresh fruit, your beautiful long fingers curved perfectly around a blueberry. I've been staring at that photo this week, losing myself in trying to get back into that moment to remember what it looked like to see you feed yourself. And sometimes I can't remember completely, and that scares me.

You haven't been sleeping well this week, and Mom and I have been taking turns being up with you. You're waking up crying, with your arms and legs tense and rigid and extended. You seem so uncomfortable. We'll rub your legs and your stomach, sway you back and forth, and eventually you'll calm back down and fall asleep on one of our shoulders or back in your rocker. But on the worst nights, which, unfortunately, have been most of them, you're up again ten minutes later. And that continues, straight on till morning, as Wendy said to Peter Pan. So this week we're facing another milestone: considering starting medication to help with your muscle tone and your sleep. I don't think we're afraid of the medication itself or even what it represents as a milestone of destructive progress. But we are afraid that the medication will sedate you and steal from us your little bit of personality,

92

of engagement, of fleeting laughter, that remains. People have warned us that these aspects of you will go away too, but it just feels too soon.

Our time back in Boston has been good to us so far. Few days have passed when there hasn't been a food delivery on the front steps: lasagna, donuts, muffins, brownies, milkshakes, smoothies, beer for Dad. So we're all eating well. And the weather has been incredible, which means lots of time outside for you which you love. Mom and I steal away for walks with you in the late afternoons and we fall in love with your dimples all over again, one stride at a time.

A little robin made its nest in a small tree off the back deck and there are three little babies chirping away to you every morning.

But even though Boston is being good to us, it feels harder to make sense of things here, where the fabric of our life before Tay-Sachs hangs in shreds on the fencepost of a milestone we passed long ago.

We love you.

Dad

* * *

In late May, Leah and Mike arrive from Dallas for a visit. Since our plan to visit them in Dallas in the middle of March was thwarted by Covid, they have not seen Havi for several months. Months is forever given Havi's condition. When they first arrive in Boston, they stay at a friend's apartment to quarantine, but they come over every day, morning and night, wearing masks and mustering up every ounce of self-restraint to not scoop Havi up and smother her with hugs and kisses.

Although Leah and Mike are masked and stand six feet away from us at all times, we relish these small family reunions. Their plan is to stay in Boston for the summer, along with Jacob and Erin, who will head east for June, July, and August. The four of them rent an apartment together. I am overjoyed that the Sibs will be a mile away from us for the next three months and amazed that they have all uprooted their lives. But according to the Sibs themselves, it makes sense for them to do this: Each of them can work remotely and none of them can imagine being away from Havi. They keep Matt and me out of all of the logistics—what it means for them to leave their homes, live with their siblings and close to their in-laws, as my parents are also moving to Boston for us, and devote themselves completely to the rhythm of our life, which is purely focused on Havi. We know they have sacrificed a lot, even though they insist that it is simple: They just want to be with Havi. It is the only place they can be.

A few days after all the Sibs arrive, my parents relocate to Boston too, leaving our family home in Philadelphia for a summer lease in a two-bedroom apartment in our neighborhood of Jamaica Plain. They make the six-hour drive to Boston in their minivan, the same one I'd grown up with, and bring my ninety-nine-year-old maternal grandfather, Zadie, along with them. They'll be right there for us, just on the other side of Jamaica Pond. Plus, my mom arranges for a new care team for Zadie through Massachusetts Veteran's Health Administration so that she can spend a few hours with Havi each day before needing to return home to full-time caregiving for her father. This extraordinary effort was simultaneously over-the-top and completely unsurprising. It's how my parents have always operated: selflessly, generously, and with an uncanny sense for showing up exactly as needed.

Now, suddenly, Matt and I are surrounded by family, and relief sets in for both of us. Havi's little sister is due to be born in June, and we know that having family close by is the only way we'll survive.

In the midst of the bizarre time of isolation created by the pandemic, Havi has brought my whole immediate family together again. After everybody completes their Covid quarantines and PCR testing, we begin gathering daily, and Havi is passed from one set of arms to another and smothered in kisses. She smiles, nuzzles, or tenderly bites a nose or a chin. And she giggles a lot this first week, everywhere, with everyone, and at the most random times.

One day, while Havi is seated in her chair at the kitchen table and I am feeding her a smoothie snack, Mike comes into the kitchen all steamed up about a difficult work phone call. He's a partner at a big-time litigation firm and is deep into preparing for a trial. As he starts to recount the details of the call to me, Havi looks up from her smoothie and laughs—a full-throated giggle bubbles up from the deepest and best of places. "Well, that call wasn't that important anyway," Mike says, and he and I both laugh along with Havi. Havi's message is simple yet wise: "Smile, Uncle Mike, don't sweat the small things, focus your energy and emotion on what really matters." We laugh and I feel lighter.

Laughter. It helps.

* * *

Havi settles easily into a summer rhythm. She is greeted by my dad, her Grandadders, every morning after one of his hot, sticky runs. My dad has always been a runner, but now he is running on behalf of Havi, so he is in "Havi Gear" now, training for his "Hav run," a seven-mile fundraising run that we are participating in on behalf of Blyth's organization, Courageous Parents Network, which takes place at the end of the summer. The fact that my dad is seventy years old doesn't matter, as he runs right alongside Matt and the Sibs and the rest of the community we have taken to calling "Havi's posse."

My dad is up and out of my parents' apartment every day before the sun rises, tracing the Boston streets and talking to Havi in his mind, for it is she who keeps him going. He tells me that running is where he puts his grief. He moves with Havi in his heart and head. Through him, I witness a grief lesson in practice: movement matters. And not as a way to "move on," rather as a way of "moving with" the hardest thing so it enhances our capacity to cope.

Grandadders comes by sweaty and breathless for a Havi kiss during breakfast before he goes home to take a shower. Then, Havi spends at least part of every day with her Grandi and Tia, and every night she has dinner with her aunts and uncles. Our table is full, our meals are long, and our sink overflows every night with dinner and dessert dishes for six. We eat every kind of vegetarian dish under the sun. We have, all six of us, committed to becoming vegetarians—the Sibs, and Matt and I—practically the day after Havi's diagnosis. It gives us a much-needed sense of control, and we love it. Except sometimes Uncle Mike sneaks a piece of peperoni pizza. But it does mean lots of black beans and lentils and other highly fibrous foods that result in, well, lots of hilariously gassy nights among six adults.

But outside our warm and loving home are violent reminders that our country is broken in many ways, that people in our country don't always show up for each other. We know this, but recent events and all-too-familiar atrocities against Black people remind us that collectively, we don't take care of each other in the ways that we should. That some human beings aren't treated as such. On May 25, George Floyd, a forty-six-year-old Black man, is murdered in Minneapolis by Derek Chauvin, a forty-four-year-old white police officer who kneels on his neck until he is unconscious—an act that a passing teenage girl captures on video and shares with the world on social media.

A few months earlier, in March, Breonna Taylor, a twenty-six-year-old Black woman, was shot and killed by the Louisville Metro Police Department during a botched no-knock warrant raid. She was not only unarmed but had been sound asleep when the police entered. And ten days before Breonna Taylor was murdered, Manuel Ellis, a thirty-three-year-old, unarmed Black man, died at the hands of the Tacoma, Washington, police force.

Then there was also Ahmaud Arbery...the list keeps going on and on.

All I can think about is all of these victims' parents. We talk about them over dinner. Then one night in early June, I listen to a podcast about George Floyd's funeral as I lie in bed with Havi. As I listen, she gazes off into the distance, as if contemplating what she hears. I respond to her intent gaze with thoughts and questions of my own—I speak them out loud to her—and she shares back with a confused look, a furrowed brow, or simply turns her head in disgust. Havi is right. None of it makes any sense. I wish more than anything that she could be a part of the next generation, the one we all hope will change and heal this country. But instead, I can't help but think about *her funeral*—how we'll endure it, what it will mean to us, and how we'll put one foot in front of the other every day afterward.

Meanwhile time is marching forward. Suddenly it is mid-June, and Father's Day is in sight. Another holiday that is meant to be celebratory. This should be among a set of first Father's Days with each of our children, featuring breakfast in bed, homemade cards, and BBQ for dinner. Instead, we will honor Matt's last Father's Day with Havi on this earth.

Our Father's Day Sunday together begins as a quiet early morning with Havi. Matt sleeps in so Havi and I surprise him with a fruit salad and challah French toast and prepare the kitchen table with gifts and decorations. I make Matt a photo album from Havi, including as many pictures of them loving up on each other as I possibly can. This album crushes Matt. "It's just too hard," he says, turning to me as he flips through the pages, "that we're actually losing her. I can't look at these." I imagine the album might have been helpful, but it isn't. And Matt looks like a shell of himself, unable to even muster up a fake smile or enjoy the challah French toast. I want to force him to talk. But I know there is really nothing for him to say. So I stop myself from pushing, and just let us be.

We move from the kitchen to the basement and finish watching *Biggest Little Farm*—a beautiful documentary that's really about the impermanence of life, and how death breeds new life. Matt and I snuggle on the couch with Havi between us. We move through the day gently, rubbing her legs during naps, and I cuddle with her in the rocking chair while Matt gets a little exercise. The house is quiet. The Sibs are giving us space. Havi and I join him for a stretch afterward, which is when Matt pops Havi into the bouncer and she giggles for what feels like eternity. We hold onto that laughter until dinnertime, when we join Grandadders and Great Zadie for a three-generation Father's Day dinner at their apartment in our neighborhood. Havi laughs again at the dinner table. Through Matt's entry, I get a window into how the day feels for him.

Hi Peanut,

I've been doing online yoga for a couple of afternoons over the last few weeks. I seem to spend most of the time sweating on the floor trying to figure out how to untangle my legs and arms from what seems to me to be some impossible contortion of the human body. And yet, surprisingly, it's felt good these past few times. But eventually comes the final shavasana relaxation and a few moments of silent reflection on the cool floor with the afternoon light filtering softly across the room. The last two times I've done yoga, the warm afternoons and their moments of quiet have reminded me of the ne'ila service at the closing of Yom Kippur, when the air feels charged with spiritual intensity. This week was no different. I closed my eyes and sank into the ground. I may have dozed off but it's hard to know. And in that moment, I saw you above me. You were older and beautiful, maybe twelve, and the afternoon light shimmered on your curls. You leaned over me and smiled and told me gently that it was time to get up. I opened my eyes. I could have touched your hand. Will you visit me like this in the future?

This week you were cute as ever and still so smiley. We seem to have figured out the right dose of your evening clonazepam. A half-tab strikes the right balance between letting you sleep all night and keeping you bright and smiley in the morning. It feels so wrong: the aluminum pill package, the white medication tablet gingerly cut into two halves, the few sips of apple juice that we sneak it into before we put you down to bed; you're too young, too sweet, too little, too cute, and too pure to have to be drugged to sleep. But we swallow hard and carry on because it keeps your restless arms and legs from jumping up uncontrollably at night and waking you. And yet your daytime naps still fall prey to the same spasticity, and every seven minutes you wake up crying hard. So for the last week there's been someone with you during almost every nap, catching your hands as your arms lock up above your head or rubbing your feet until your eyelids droop and you fall back to sleep.

But on the cute side of things, you officially outgrew your eighteen-month sleeping onesies, which meant a migration to a new set of twenty-four-months-sized adorable PJs. So each night and every morning is a fashion show of cuteness, not that we need a reminder of how beautiful you are.

The step-by-step chronicle of how we're losing you is sometimes too crushing. We're grasping on to the littlest things, to keep as much of you with us for as long as we can.

"Is she still laughing?" my dad asked one day when I was talking to him on the phone. "Yeah," I said, and nearly threw the phone through the glass window I was standing next to. When does the answer become "no"? How many more days do we have?

While I was working today, your mom texted me a photo of you with your Uncle Jacob on the back deck. I was at work when the photo came through. You were cradled in his arms and he smiled at you with the purest expression of complete delight. Your blond curls dangled beautifully behind your head and you looked up at him. The photo stopped me; it reminded me of another photo of you and Uncle Jacob, taken in nearly the same spot, almost a year ago to the day. In that photo the two of you sit on the ground, facing each other, and your uncle looks down at you and you gaze back at him, your eyes bright, and you have the cutest smile, showing off your little dimples.

You were sitting up on your own when that picture was taken, and with the most perfect posture and strongest core and a confident gaze in your eyes. There were no signs then of what lay ahead for you. These two photos, side-by-side, make me think about a few things. The first is that you have so much more story than just the last twenty-seven Shabbirthdays. You rolled over, and crawled, and fed yourself blueberries, and stood in your crib and babbled at us like any healthy little baby. That time, when things were "normal," is part of your story too and we need to tell it and share it. And the second thing is that the photo of you with your Uncle Jacob last year made me realize that despite your changes, despite the disease that is stealing you from us every day, the love you have generated and the love that you receive is no different today than it was before. In fact, it's even grown.

I got a text message yesterday from a friend saying, "Happy Father's Day!" I had forgotten, or maybe I put it out of my mind. My thoughts swirled: Do I even want to celebrate this? Do I hate Father's Day? How do you even begin to celebrate your last Father's Day with your child? I have no fucking idea how to navigate that. Every day counts now, not just the third Sunday in June.

You gave me the best Father's Day gift, though. You laughed harder and longer than you ever have. I popped you in the bouncer that we used in your much earlier days and slowly rocked you back and forth. You smiled, then you cooed, and then you giggled and what followed can only be described as unrestrained howling laughter for over ten minutes. You anticipated my touch and you asked for more with every squeal.

We love you.

Dad

CHAPTER 20

Kaia Lev

The next morning, we jump back into the work week. Like always, we hang on tightly to the moments between Zoom calls when we join Havi for a meal, steal a few kisses from her, or whisper "I love you" in her ear. That morning, I also have a chance to cuddle with Havi in her bedroom in the white rocking chair to talk about the impending arrival of her baby sister. Each time I bring the new baby up, she wraps her arms around my neck, bends her knees and hips, sticks out her butt and squats down on the top of my pregnant belly, lifting her chest and holding her head high to nuzzle into my neck.

Somehow her movements seem bigger and stronger today, at least in my mind, and I even let myself imagine she is beating Tay-Sachs. I run my hands through her curls and tell myself, *She's doing it. She's going to be the first person to ever overcome this horrible disease. And she'll share her tricks with anyone who ever has to endure this.* But then she startles and spasms and pulls me back to reality. I guess that every parent feels at some point like their child has some kind of superpower. I only wish that overcoming Tay-Sachs could have been Havi's.

Maybe her unusual strength this day is in response to the joyful news that her little sister will arrive soon. We spend some time preparing for the new baby's arrival, but I feel fear creeping into my body and have a hard time participating in preparing her room. Matt takes the lead.

I am big now, and can feel my body preparing to give birth. I want to talk to Havi about the new baby, about how some of our routines will change, and get her input on her little sister's name. Mostly, though, I worry. What if the testing is wrong again? What if we aren't meant to parent living children? Our parenting naivete has been shattered. And yet, I know that, just as it is with loving Havi, loving our new baby will be fully worth the risk of losing her. Opening myself up to more love and more loss is scary as hell.

Havi's little sister will only know Havi through us, so Matt and I promise each other that we will be strong for that reason. Also, we promise to recognize our newborn as a completely unique and beautiful being. She will also carry pieces of Havi. Through our new baby, we'll also come to know Havi differently.

This is not how I ever expected our family to expand, and I wish it could be very, very different for both of the girls. Havi's sister will know too much loss. She'll have to carry that with her for a lifetime.

*   *   *

Then, very suddenly, although we have been awaiting her for a long time, Kaia is born. The details are blurry to me, although I do remember Havi's gentle hands guiding her down the birth canal. Matt captures my missing recollections in his entry this week.

> Hi Peanut,
>
> This was a pretty big week. On Monday morning, after your mom and I made a few calls, feigning the beginning of a regular workweek, your mom went into labor with your baby sister. We had prepared for this day, maybe a little later than would be ideal, but we had everything you needed ready. We'd outfitted your little sister's bedroom and transcribed your smoothie recipes for your Grandi, Aunt Leah, and Tia to follow to the letter. Aunt Leah had even written down every word of our nightly bedtime routine, from saying goodnight to the bay all the way to singing Eric Clapton's "Wonderful Tonight" and "Have I Told You Lately" to you as you drift off—as your mom and I do every night. So with all that complete, and your mom's contractions starting, we packed a small bag, said goodbye to you for the first time since getting your diagnosis seven months ago, and headed off to the Brigham.
>
> By now it feels like we've been to the Brigham too many times, so the emotional weight of the turn we take onto

Francis Street forces your mom and me to retreat into silence every time. There was an impossible, indescribable mix of anticipatory excitement and heartbreaking sadness heavy in the humid air as we pulled into a parking space.

Mom got checked in at the labor and delivery desk and I waited outside with our bag. The hum of hospital business seemed no different than my first days of residency. An excited, nervous-looking couple sat in chairs a few feet away from me, and I felt like I was looking into a snow globe of our prior life. We made it upstairs and into our room as the afternoon light started to illuminate the collection of building angles and edges outside our window. It was quiet, and the nurses gave us our space. And in a few hushed moments it was just your mom and me, together again, alone, sitting a few inches apart from one another, and talking about everything and nothing.

We discovered that my shorts had a hole in the crotch so we perused a few online stores and ordered a new pair. Then we excitedly reviewed the hospital food menu; our "regular diet" order allowed us nearly free reign except for a head-scratching restriction on ordering milkshakes, which left me quite displeased. Needless to say, we ordered dinner twice and nibbled on awful but still somehow delicious and satisfying hospital meals. For a moment in that quiet room, we felt safe, isolated, protected. It made me realize how painful it is sometimes to exist in this world, to navigate old spaces feeling like a ghost.

At some point the light turned to dusk and Mom's breathing changed. For a while I just watched her as she calmly rolled in and out of contractions, a few long strands of her rich, brown hair having come loose from her hair tie, falling gently past her ear. She's so beautiful, your mom, which I know you already know, but there was something especially beautiful about her then. I tried to be of some service, but like I do at her marathons, I mostly just cheered her on.

It didn't help that I was having my own regular contractions—of the GI kind, thanks to the black bean burger in dinner No. 1. "Seriously, Emmy?!?!" she'd say. "Now?!?" So maybe I was less than helpful. But still, we danced, she pressed her head into my chest, squeezed my hand, and with a single push, your sister was born. Your mom never broke a sweat. No pain meds. Instead, thinking of you was the antidote for her painful contractions and I know that helped bring Kaia safely into our world.

Kaia Lev Goldstein. Your little sister. She weighed in at 6 lb. 12 oz.—just a little bigger than you; you were 6 lb. 9 oz. Kaia was 19 inches long; you were 18.75 inches. Kaia's fingers are long like yours—both of you have hands like your mom's—and you and Kaia were both demonstrably strong the moment you arrived. Also, it seems that you both, also just like your mom, get the hiccups an inordinate amount. The other day, home from the hospital, we placed photos we'd taken of each of you, at just a couple days old, side-by-side, and they are nearly identical. (We put them into a frame; you're the one on the left, by the way.)

You and Kaia share a middle name, Lev, meaning "heart" in Hebrew, and your first names come from the same Hebrew root, chai, meaning life. Life and love. That's what you both are and will always be for us and for this entire community that has come to know and love you. You and Kaia are the two most closely related humans on this planet, and when we lose you, we will still have a part of you through Kaia. On the morning we got home from the hospital we sat her next to you. We placed your arm around Kaia's neck and she rolled toward you, onto your shoulder. With your other arm, you reached for her thigh. Your bond is strong.

You look so big, so wise, so poised and mature. And you're not even two years old yet, and you're dying. There are too many thoughts crowding into my mind, Hav. There are too many moments when a look, a startle, a laugh, or a smile send a cascade of the most complex emotions rippling through me to lodge heavily in the middle of my chest.

Since December 17, your diagnosis day, I've wanted to cherish, capture, hold onto every moment with you. Now that Kaia is here, that feels even more pressing. We're a family of four now, and you're a beautiful older sister, exactly as I expected you to be, and yet Tay-Sachs—fuck that disease—is simultaneously trying to erase you from the future of our story. But Mom and I will never let you be erased, for the record, even though there is no space in this universe that can encompass the void that we will feel when you are gone.

You turned twenty-two months old today. Yesterday was your twenty-ninth Shabbirthday and the first one we celebrated with your baby sister, Kaia Lev. You're surrounded and kissed and hugged and showered, nearly every moment of every day, with love. We were in the hospital, away from you, for forty-eight hours, and I missed you so much that I sobbed into your shoulder when we got home.

How will we be away from you forever one day?

We love you so much.

Dad

* * *

Kaia moves into our third bedroom upstairs, and our house is wonderfully full. I love walking past the girls' bedrooms on the way to mine and Matt's, knowing that our two girls are only steps away from us and from each other. We settle quickly into a routine. Maybe it is the controlled chaos of having a newborn in the house or perhaps we'd just found some sort of rhythm that, for a few weeks at least, makes us feel like we can be any young family on the block.

Every morning, when Matt turns off the sound machine that we keep in Havi's room to calm her at night, she rocks her head back and forth and smiles during the first few weeks of Kaia's life. And during these weeks Havi's appetite is particularly robust, not uncoincidentally timed with a real step-up in our smoothie game: blueberry muffins, peanut butter, oat milk, avocado, and vanilla protein powder. She weighs twenty-three pounds, shattering her previous weight.

It seems so suddenly she has become the older sister I imagined she would be. And, it is a good thing too, because baby Kaia is really putting us through our paces with a continuum of crying, grunting, spitting up, pooping, peeing, and pooping again. Through dinner, Havi sits quietly and calmly in her chair, waiting for Matt or me to soothe her, and then greets us with big eyes and a big open-mouthed smile when we sit back down next to her. It's as if, in her precocious wisdom, she knows everything that is going on. I wonder if I am imposing that sense of astuteness on her, and I embrace it anyway. I'm allowed. Anyway, I suppose I could be guilty of under-estimating it, too. So, why not trust my feelings.

When we are out walking with the girls, or on Zoom calls, sometimes we encounter people who don't understand the full extent of the Tay-Sachs diagnosis and they exclaim that Havi must be so excited to have her little sister here. I always agree that, yes, Havi is excited about Kaia, and then I change the subject to some standard topic regarding newborns, like sleep cycles or eating patterns. The truth is, I don't know any more what Havi understands about Kaia or anything else, and it slays me to go down the path of trying to answer that question. We have been living in a bubble, as Charlie and Blyth call it, and I am fine existing in that place where Havi's moments are magnified, where her little sounds seem to unfold into conversations about our days and her eyes radiate with the joy of having a table full of people celebrating her over dinner.

Outside of the bubble can be hurtful. In fact, one day we have a short call with our lawyer that reinforces this. The conversation is cold and calculated. As we do the dishes that night, Matt turns to me and says that his feelings about the lawsuit are all mixed up and complicated: On the one hand, it is a way for us to feel like we are parenting Havi, or at least defending her to a system that has failed her in the most significant way. On the other hand, it captures the worst parts of medicine. The current "cover your ass" guideline-driven system of care leaves out all the most important things that make doctors, healers. Everyone acknowledges the error that led to Havi being born with Tay Sachs, but we still struggle and battle through every call to justify why a system change is needed. "Isn't it obvious?" Matt says he sometimes finds himself wanting to scream.

Having finished drying the last plate, he throws the dishtowel on the counter, and says, "I need some air. Taking a walk."

CHAPTER 21

Dr. Jo

July 18, 2020. Havi is twenty-two months old.
"It's a tragic privilege to know you," Dr. Jo says. "I wish you didn't have to know me." Matt and I are sitting on our back deck, my cell phone on the table between us, taking our first call with the revered grief therapist Dr. Joanne Cacciatore. Dr. Jo is ours for an hour every other week, thanks to Aunt Erin, who gifted us these sessions.

"I can't cure your grief. Nor would we want that," Dr. Jo says. "Grieving is a form of loving Havi. Loving everything you have with her, and every moment you won't have."

Immediately I feel safe with Dr. Jo. "I think we've found our person," I say to Matt when the session ends. Matt nods. "I think we have."

* * *

Matt and I meet with Dr. Jo by phone once every two weeks. Mostly, we take her calls in Havi's room. Her soft, comforting voice sounds like a smile. Once we've said our hellos, and she's asked about Havi, she takes a deep, slow breath. Reflexively, we do too: a deep inhalation followed by a long, audible exhalation. Then we're ready to talk.

"Where is your grief living today?"

I start. "It's in my throat. Sometimes I swallow a few times to make sure I still can. And then I wonder why I get to swallow if Havi won't be able to at some point."

Jo says, "It's cellular, isn't it? The pain and the love of a mother."

"Yes. And I've been clenching my fists a lot too, which is new."

"I've heard that from a lot of parents. I wonder if it is a demonstration of an inner-protestation: How could this be?"

Matt jumps in. "I've been in a state of disbelief. So that resonates."

"Yes," Jo agrees. "Disbelief is merciful. Gives us time to move mountains one stone at a time."

Wow, I think. I love that. In unison, Matt and I each take a deep breath. Feeling safe makes it so much easier to breathe.

Dr. Jo lost her daughter too. She knows the depths of our grief. She also has twenty-five years of experience working with families like ours, while teaching her students at Arizona State University about the complexity and anguish of losing a child. In our conversations with her, it's always okay to feel what we're feeling: anguish, numbness, fear, despair, anger, impatience, withdrawal. "As we work with our feelings," she tells us, "they become conscious. Then we can trust them."

"Your loss, your tragedy is abnormal," she says. "Your feelings are not."

Dr. Jo ends every call with the same words. "Give that beautiful girl a kiss from her friend in Arizona."

* * *

Every couple days, I pull dozens of Havi's bibs from the washing machine and transfer them to the dryer. Her drooling is causing her to soak through a bib an hour. Our beautiful girl is changing in heartbreaking ways. She's laughing less. Her exaggerated startle response means the creak of a floorboard or the click of a door latch wakes her, and it's getting harder for her to fall back to sleep. It takes us massaging her arms, her legs, and her feet to calm her. We've turned her sound machine up so high, she wouldn't hear a rock concert in the room next door.

One morning Aunt Leah spends two and a half hours helping Havi take a nap so Matt and I can sleep. Later, she tells us that Havi needed another massage every seven minutes. Havi is choking on her saliva more often.

We have a bottle of pills to ease these side-effects. We keep it, unopened, on the kitchen counter. That medication makes Havi even sleepier during the day, and we don't want her to miss out on anything during her precious remaining days. Matt and I make the judgment call that as long as Havi's eyes are open, she's enjoying what's left of her life.

In recent weeks and months, as the pandemic continues to rage, family and friends would Covid-cautiously arrive in Boston Airbnbs, and gaze in at Havi and Kaia through our living room windows.

On Havi's thirty-first Shabbirthday, Grandma and Grandpa, visiting from California, are finally able to cross the threshold into our house. Kelsey and her boyfriend also drove up from New York. The Sibs meander over from their new Boston summer residence. Then, like a scene straight out of a Disney movie, balloons, trays of food, and bottles of wine march through our front door, courtesy of Matt's company. With our plates piled high and our glasses filled, we toast Havi and Kaia.

CHAPTER 22

Walks

Havi's thirty-first Shabbirthday is magical, but the next Shabbirthday is the one that Erin calls *our nightmare dream*. We celebrate Havi's thirty-second Shabbirthday over pizza and beer, with our entire family at the table, including Aunt Maggie, who has just flown in from Colorado. It feels like a dream that we are all together, and yet it turns into a nightmare when we begin talking openly about why we have to celebrate so hard every Friday night.

The next day I sit in the white rocker in Havi's room with the shades drawn. The afternoon light slides in around the window's edges as she lies across my legs, taking a nap. Her head tilts toward my body so I have a perfect view of her face. Her eyes are closed and her impossibly long and dark lashes curl outward as always. Her expression is peaceful, tender, and innocent. She looks like an angel. *She is an angel.* Her beauty moves me to tears.

I cry as I peer down at her because I am in a quiet room with time and space to think. My mind comes to rest on the fact that she is dying and I can't will her back to health. Too soon, I'll have to close my eyes and *imagine* she is lying across me because she won't *be* with me, the warmth of her skin will be gone, out of reach. It is the finality of her eventual death that scares me most. Death. The only thing that is permanent. I don't know what to do with these thoughts, where to put them, and so I cry. I sit watching her, studying her, and loving her. Being with the pain keeps me in my body and I notice how it changes even over five minutes.

Just a few feet away from Havi, Kaia sleeps too. The two nap together as often as possible. That's how each of them spends a lot of the day, so it feels like the best way for them to bond, to know each other's sounds and scents. Maybe it is my imagination, but it seems like Havi sleeps better when Kaia is in the room. Kaia seems to soften Havi's startles, stabilizing her the way any good sister does. And sometimes I will see Havi looking down on Kaia, seeming to offer the sort of unspoken, admiring love that only a sister can give.

On several mornings during these first weeks of Kaia's life, we take walks as a family of four. Kaia is in the carrier against Matt's chest as I push Havi in the stroller. Matt walks with his cup of coffee, and I hold my tea, each of our mugs with a V-shaped crack at the rim from many mornings of good use—cracked but still functioning, like us. They are beautiful, handmade ceramic mugs from Dirt Cowboy, our favorite coffee shop on Dartmouth's campus. As we take our walk this morning, I think deeply about the day when Matt asks me to marry him, at Dartmouth— and how after he proposed, we held each other, and kissed, and held each other some more. And how all I could say afterward was, "Our kids will not be going to private school."

Matt laughed and said, "You're a nut, but whatever you want, baby." He had gone to private school, and for some reason I had developed a thing against such places. Really, it was totally unfounded, and I'd come to a much more sophisticated view of education over the years, but at that moment, I had skipped ahead about a hundred steps in our life. I guess my protesting private school was my crazy way of saying that I wanted to have a family with Matt. I also wanted our family to avoid being caught up in an elite world that didn't feel good or right.

Eventually, I would have to undo all that sort of thinking. Matt and I would come to understand this sort of future planning was, in many ways, futile, along with the idea that you have any control over what's ahead.

Then Havi startles awake and I am brought back to the present, to our taking a walk down May Street just a few blocks from home.

Whenever Havi starts to cry on these walks, I lean over and mas- sage her legs and kiss her cheeks as we wind our way up toward Moss Hill. Meanwhile, Kaia sleeps soundly against Matt's chest. Matt and I can't help but comment on how different Havi's experience was from Kaia's. At Kaia's age, Havi just couldn't get comfortable in the carrier. We'd tried everything—brought along a sound machine on our walks to block out noise, splurged on a "better" carrier, timed our walks to fit per- fectly between feeds and naps—and still Havi couldn't settle, and we had thought that was normal.

We used to marvel at the young families who bounced between shops with a baby sleeping soundly in a carrier. "Maybe she just wants to be able to see the world," we'd say to each other. "Maybe we have the wrong kind of carrier." So many rationalizations for what turns out to be Tay-Sachs.

Now I am sorry for all the times we had put Havi in an uncomfortable position. And yet, as her Uncle Jacob says, Havi is "perhaps best described in three words: beauty, grace, and toughness." We walk together as a family of four. Matt greets every breeze by spreading his arms wide, standing tall with his chest puffed with pride, smiling broadly, and saying, "Hi, sweet girl, Hi Hav." Other walkers pass by and smile at us. They have no idea. No one really ever does know what's going on inside someone else's life.

CHAPTER 23

Seizure

It is August now and one Sunday morning we can tell it is going to be another hot day. The early morning sun filters in through the kitchen skylight. Havi sits in her chair at the kitchen table slurping on a smoothie of kale, avocado, and mango with a spoonful of Miralax. Upstairs, Kaia still sleeps. The outside world is quiet. Only the birds are awake.

Matt and I sit on either side of Havi, and the two of us huddle close to her. I hold her head, and Matt holds her bottle, navigating the straw carefully in between her tightly locked lips. Havi's arms rest on the table in front of her, her hands held in tight little fists. The morning light streams across her face, bringing her light eyes and red lips into focus. Stevie Nicks' "Landslide" plays in the background, and I notice tears streaming down Matt's face. He sings this to Havi almost every day for the first year of her life. She is calmed as he sings these lyrics, holding her body curled up against his chest, the two of them swaying gently together. "Landslide" evokes both the natural world and a father-daughter relationship for us, and I know that for the rest of my life, hearing it will always make me think of Havi and Matt.

I reach across Havi to wipe Matt's tears from his cheek, and my heart breaks. Seeing Matt aching is the hardest thing, one of the cruelest aspects of Havi's disease.

Charlie and Blyth bring bagels and pastries for Sunday brunch. They meet my parents for the first time. We all sit in the kitchen, smearing extra cream cheese on our bagels, eating one too many rugelach, and passing Havi from one lap to another. Kaia naps upstairs in her crib. I hear her stir and I pop upstairs to feed her. After I finish feeding Kaia, kiss her fiercely, and put her back to sleep, I walk downstairs. I hear the hum of quiet conversation and smell coffee and bagels. I think to myself, this is a beautiful way to spend a Sunday morning.

But as I enter the room, Blyth catches my gaze and, with tears in her eyes, shares what had happened: "Havi just had a seizure," she says with a tenderness in her voice. "Are you sure? How do you know?"

"Yes, sweetie. I am sure. Her arm shook, her neck tensed, a clicking hum pulsed repeatedly from her mouth, and then she seemed far away. It wasn't very long. Maybe fifteen seconds. And she was on my lap. Comfortable."

Blyth is still holding Havi, but hands her to me. Havi falls asleep almost immediately in my arms. "They can be very tiring. I wouldn't be surprised if she sleeps more today than usual," Blyth adds.

I sit, holding sleeping Havi, Matt pulls up a chair next to me, and Charlie and Blyth talk us through what just happened: an inevitable but still incomprehensible transition in the arc of her story. "She's not in any pain," Charlie reassures us. "When it happens again, massage the soft area between her thumb and index finger; that helps," Blyth explains.

I sit, jiggling my legs and knocking my knees together. I bite my quivering lip and turn into Blyth's shoulder. I let myself cry into her sweater. She knows loss as a mother. I need her strength.

It is a gift that they are with us when Havi's first seizure happens. The mystery of our friendship continues to astound me. That on this morning, Havi and Blyth find their way to each other, so that Blyth can literally hold us as we witness our daughter's first seizure—an explicit, dramatic signal that Havi's central nervous system is failing her. Her body seizes and shakes until she sleeps from exhaustion. We are shaken by reality; Blyth provides equilibrium. Friendships that work, that operate on a level above any sense of obligation or necessity, that are beyond description, that show up when you need them—we miraculously and mysteriously inherited one of those.

I'd seen seizures before in movies. They are scary and unsettling. But in a few more scenes, life always seems to return to normal. Most often, there is some happy ending. But we would have no happy ending. So, later that day, we walk upstairs to our bathroom, accompanied by Grandi and Grandadders and the Sibs, and pull out the basket of medications we've accumulated. We haven't yet opened the thin, rectangular box holding Havi's prescription for rectal Valium, which we filled before leaving for the Havimoon. The doctors called it "rescue medicine." Inside the box are two small packets of lubricating gel, two syringes, and an instruction pamphlet, featuring cartoon images, like the ones on the emergency safety cards stuffed into the backs of seats on airplanes. We spread everything out on the bathroom counter. We know that in case Havi's seizures intensify or begin lasting longer than five minutes, we will need to use Valium, so everyone in our house needs to know how to administer it. As I read the instructions aloud to our family, I catch a glimpse of Matt and me in the bathroom mirror. *Help*, I want to say to my reflection. *How did we get here?*

*   *   *

I hope against hope that Havi's seizure that Sunday is a single event, but as the weeks roll on, one seizure becomes two, two becomes three, and soon I lose count.

Just about every morning, as Matt and I huddle close to Havi, feeding her a smoothie and kissing her cheeks, her arms start to shake and her fingers stiffen. Her neck tightens and her head angles awkwardly. She makes a quiet but strange sound, over and over and over. Her eyes become distant. Matt massages her hand between her thumb and index finger, as Charlie and Blyth instructed us. We sit still and quiet, just waiting. Then the seizure stops. Even though each seizure only lasts about fifteen seconds, it always feels like forever. This is our new normal? Her new normal. I can't protect my child. What the fuck.

Later that day, Matt and I need to get out of the house, and we also need a loaf of bread for dinner, so we leave Havi and Kaia with their two aunts and uncles and drive to the grocery store. But we drive in silence, Matt's hand on mine. At the store, we walk around in a daze. Somehow all of the food is making us feel nauseous. Not even the ice cream looks good.

I want to roll back time to a different series of firsts, to Havi's first smile, her first coo, the first time she rolled over, her first solid food, our first trip with her on an airplane. Her life seemed like it was going to be so vast and mysterious and wonderful. We didn't know who she'd become, but we'd be along for the ride. And now all of that is gone, lost in the corner of our kitchen counter that is piled with syringes, pills, and liquid medications. We are caught in a war between sedation and seizures, hoping that both sides lose. Havi is slouching more and having a harder time holding her head up. I can feel her physical being fighting to stay present, to stay here with us. Follow her lead, I tell myself as I sleep walk through the grocery store. Somehow, Matt finds the bread. We drive home.

Kaia's big smile greets us when we walk through the door. She is beginning her own list of milestones. She slipped out her first smile this past week. She is becoming more alert, focused, and interested in the world around her. Just as Havi begins to turn inward, to cocoon, Kaia is turning outward, expanding her world. As Havi needs more sleep and quiet, Kaia craves stimulation. At times, the contrast is stark and hard to watch, but at other moments it seems like a beautiful dance to which only the two of them know the steps. I feel the bond growing between them, as I watch Kaia focus her eyes on Havi's and reach her arms toward her big sister. At some point in the near future, that bond will have to stretch through the veil between the worlds of the living and the dead. But in the meantime, Havi seems to be getting a massive kick out of Kaia's squawking escapades, and Kaia is drawn to her big sister's calm, tender presence.

Kaia's smiles and demands help us have the strength to deal with Havi's postictal state, the altered state of consciousness that follow a seizure, which is characterized by drowsiness, confusion, nausea, and headaches.

And Havi is stretching us to hold everything—not only the cruel injustice of Tay-Sachs, but also the compassion, courage, and kindness that exist just beyond the disease. And that stretching hurts and also makes day-to-day living harder. We decide we need a change of scene.

CHAPTER 24

The Ocean

After almost six months without any interaction with the real world beyond my immediate family, I decide to plan our first family road trip—to a lovely inn in Chatham on Cape Cod for two days, just a two-hour drive away, with the Sibs and my parents. Matt and I promise to get Havi back to the water, and Matt's birthday, August 12, seems like the opportunity for us to make good on that promise. We book our rooms at the last minute and squeeze in our stay by the sea just before the seven-mile Courageous Parents Network fundraising run that we'd all participate in when we return to Boston.

Leah and I write up a packing list for Havi: four pre-made smoothies to cover the two full days away, a stack of bibs and burp cloths, old medications, new medications, the rescue medication, baby seat, towels we use to keep her head propped up at all her meals, and a bathing suit of course. I am excited about going away, but as I zip up the luggage, I suddenly feel nervous about leaving. Havi hasn't been having a particularly good time lately. Her new seizure medication makes her sleepy and she can't seem to stay awake for more than an hour anymore before she needs another nap. Her eyes aren't as bright as before and her smiles have been reduced to mere hints of expression at the corners of her mouth. But most distressing is her loss of appetite. Though I sit with Havi at the table for hours, trying to get her to eat, she barely finishes an ounce of her smoothie. Our neurologist doesn't seem to think that it could be medication related so Matt and I begin to wonder, with tightened chests, whether this too, is a new phase in her disease.

But I remember our values. Be with people we love. Get Havi and Kaia to beautiful places together. Relinquish control. Maybe the trip will do Havi good, since she has always loved the ocean. Plus, the weather is hot, and we are booked to go, and we'd have the whole family with us for support. So I swallow my uncertainty and help bring the luggage out to the car.

We leave early in the morning on the day after Matt's birthday, trying to time the girls' naps for the car ride. Leah, Erin, Jacob, and Grandadders follow us to Chatham. In our car, Grandi rides in the front with Matt while I sit in the back seat, wedging myself in between Havi and Kaia's car seats, keeping a hand on each of them the whole way. Fortunately, they both fall asleep before we leave the driveway. After about thirty minutes, Havi wakes up and looks at me. She is very alert, as if she knows we are headed somewhere good.

Though it is still early morning when we arrive in Chatham, the heat has already wrapped itself around everything. As soon as we settle into our rooms, we walk together down to the sea, where the lightest breeze, blowing off the water, plays with Havi's golden curls. She tips her head back, opens her mouth wide, and lets the salt air wash deep into her lungs. Now her eyes sparkle again, and she stays awake all afternoon to take in our beautiful spot. Kaia sleeps peacefully in the carrier against my chest for most of the afternoon. Each of our girls loves being by the water.

*　*　*

The next morning, as we meander toward the dining room for breakfast, a family of four walks toward us, all wearing matching Native-brand beach shoes. I catch Matt looking intently at their feet as we pass them, and I know his mind is accelerating through a swirling wormhole of moments, memories, and images of the future we would not have with Havi. He had bought Havi two pairs of those same shoes sometime around her first birthday—he couldn't decide between the yellow and the gray so he bought them both. They wound up being too big at the time, and then, by the time Havi had grown enough to wear them, she wasn't walking anyway. We pulled them out again several months later when we needed a wider shoe to fit around the ankle and foot orthotics—leg braces—that Havi was fitted for to help her stand. Matt made two small cuts on either side of the shoes to make them easier to get on and off around the rigid plastic brace. But she only wore the braces once, and she hated them, and soon after that she was diagnosed with Tay-Sachs, so the braces and the shoes had been sitting unused in the corner of her room ever since. Matt doesn't say a word, but his energy shifts. I know just where he is.

We spend Havi's thirty-fifth Shabbirthday at the beach. After looking at Matt like he is nuts to bring her into the less-than-warm water, she happily kicks her legs around in it. Kaia sleeps in the carrier against my chest, occasionally lifting her head and opening her eyes wide to take in the scene. We are careful to keep her fully covered to protect her newborn skin from the summer sun. I like having Kaia against my chest. I feel like I can keep her safe. Later, as Matt and the girls and I sit under an umbrella and watch the waves, the most delicious breeze blows past as if saying hi to our sweetest little peas. Havi dozes and then, as the sun plays on the waves, she takes a deep breath and sighs as if to say, *Took you long enough to get us back to the beach, guys.*

We all eat dinner on the patio outside our room overlooking the beach and about a dozen small sailboats moored a short distance from shore. The sky is blue, then yellow, then pink, then lavender and the afternoon breeze has found its way to evening. We sit after eating, talking about the sunset when a little giggle tumbles out of Havi's mouth and catches us all by surprise. We turn toward her, our conversation pauses, and we wait, hoping that her sweet giggle will come again. And it does. Listen for laughter.

On our last morning by the sea, Matt and I take Havi for a walk along a stone pathway, past wispy sea grasses and hydrangeas in full bloom, to the ocean for one last inhale of the moist, salty air that she loves. Everybody else, Kaia included, waits for us back at the inn. Now that she is six weeks old Kaia is beginning to make real eye contact, and she already has her aunts and uncles and grandparents wrapped around her little finger.

Down on the beach, storm clouds gather, signaling to Matt and me that it is almost time to leave, so we park Havi's stroller near two big rocks and sit on them next to her, facing the water. We meditate. Dr. Jo introduced us to the practice, teaching us the importance of being where our feet are, and fully taking in all the smells, sights, and sounds to give us the best chance of remembering. During one early call, Dr. Jo shared a concept that evolved into another lesson: There is no safe-distance to loving. In fact, keeping feelings at a distance can strain our bodies and close our hearts. Trying to distance ourselves from pain and heartache will only cause more damage. "Love Havi fully today," Dr. Jo told us, "and after she dies."

Every few breaths I turn to look at Havi, to "paint" over her features with my eyes, tracing them again and again and again, trying to memorize them. Then I turn away and close my eyes, picture her face in my mind, and then open my eyes again to test myself. I check to see if my memory had gotten it right. Are her lips really that cherry red, and her eyes really such a deep green-gold? Maybe if I close my eyes tightly enough and work hard enough, the shape of her nose, the smell of her hair, the touch of her cheek against mine will be just as true later in my life as they are in this moment.

Then, just after I reopen my eyes, Havi stirs in her stroller. Another spasm overtakes her. Suddenly her legs are straight with her long, fine, ballerina-shaped toes pointed tautly toward the water, and her whole body extends. A low cry rises from her lips. I hate this part. Matt and I stand up, massage her feet and legs until it is over, and then walk slowly back to our car, where Kaia and the rest of our family waits for us.

Kaia cries the whole way home. Remarkably, Havi sleeps through most of Kaia's fussing. She startles awake at a sniffle or at a creak in the floor, but whenever Kaia cries, her lips turn upward to form a quiet smile and she sighs and stays asleep.

CHAPTER 25

Running Time

We make it home in time for the fundraiser's pre-race pasta dinner, and then tuck ourselves into bed early. Sunday morning arrives quickly. Race day. We are all running seven miles to raise money for the Courageous Parents Network, Blyth's organization that supports families like ours. I promised to get my run in early, and then stay with Havi and Kaia during the actual race. So Matt and I tag-team on morning duties—administering medicine, changing diapers, packing burp cloths. After I breastfeed Kaia, I lace up my sneakers and hit the pavement at 6:00 a.m.

It is quiet and cool and the streets are empty. I run my own course through the neighborhoods I normally walk with Havi. Then I hit the dirt paths through the bucolic Allandale Farm, and head back toward home. I pass several spots that are loaded with beautiful and painful memories of Havi—the park where we held her baby shower two years earlier, as well as through some neighborhoods where we imagined moving when Havi was old enough for kindergarten. While my legs turn quickly, I soar through memories of her. Seven miles later, I am home. I take a long, deep breath before opening the front door, and wonder how I'll walk through this door after she dies.

My family's pre-race jitters are palpable when I walk back in the front door. Havi sits with Matt at the kitchen table, wearing her all-black race-day uniform while she slurps her smoothie, kicking her legs beneath the table, and looking deeply into Matt's eyes, as if to say, *You can do it, Dad. I'll be waiting for you at the finish.* On my way upstairs to the shower, I hear the sounds of the rest of our family, who'd come over early, scurrying around the house making final preparations—filling water bottles, repeating visits to the bathroom, and changing outfits. I spot Matt's all-black race-day uniform matching Havi's laid out on our bed. He's such a gear guy. I smile.

Soon we load Havi and Kaia into the car and head for Charlie and Blyth's house. There is a small group gathered there: parents who have lost children, providers who work in palliative care, and various friends and supporters. We stand in a circle in Charlie and Blyth's backyard, and all introduce ourselves and share why we are running. "For Havi," Matt and my dad and I say. Then I add, "And for every family who faces this impossible journey." I mean it. But I look across the circle at mothers who have lost their children and I want to run away. I don't want to be them. And I hate myself for that thought.

I bring Havi and Kaia with us as everyone moves from the backyard to the starting line, and we watch as ten runners from Havi's posse head for Heartbreak Hill, the iconic Boston marathon hill which makes or breaks a runner. The weather is perfect for a run: in the sixties and over-cast, with a gentle Havi breeze of course.

After spending some time with Blyth, I walk to a nice spot around mile-marker 6.5 to cheer on our family members. It is a seven-mile race, and one by one, they come pounding down Cotton Road, each one accelerating the instant they see Havi and Kaia. They all have an extra bounce in their step and a wider smile than I'd seen in a long time, as if they could run forever, and I know why. The race ends with long, emotional embraces and lots of happy and sad tears. Taylor, Charlie and Blyth's oldest daughter, designed the perfect seven-mile loop. Running has a new meaning in our lives now, all wrapped up with therapeutic purpose and rage and heartbreak and healing. None of us knows where running will take us, but we'll all make sure to have Havi's spirit with us for every stride.

Matt and I sleep hard that night and wake up early Monday morn-ing in time for a virtual meeting with Havi's feeding specialist, Amanda Hull. Unlike many of our interactions with the medical world, talking to Amanda feels good. She makes Havi's life better by helping to preserve her independence and maintain her blueberry muffin intake, and she always treats Havi like the beautiful toddler she is. But this meeting feels different because we have to discuss the seizures and what they mean.

I hesitate before asking, "Are we reaching the end of the road here?"

"Yes, you are," Amanda says softly but firmly. "The next stage is cup feeding when you'll slowly pour Havi's smoothie in her mouth. Keep her drinking from the straw as long as you can."

Even Amanda is running out of tricks. After we end the session, Matt and I cry. Food is such a fundamental part of life—especially for Havi. She loves food, and our meals together define much of our time with her, and now Tay-Sachs is taking that away too.

CHAPTER 26

The Sibs

The Sibs' summer rental ends in a month, and they spend several weekends touring Boston rentals as a group of four adults, meeting realtors who would inevitably look at them somewhat cross-eyed when they explain that Jacob and Leah are brother and sister and Erin and Mike are their respective spouses, and that the four of them are looking to cohabitate in Boston for a while. Jacob tells us sometimes they even bring Havi and/or Kaia with them, and when a realtor says, "Your daughters are beautiful," they simply say, "Thank you." In fact, on any given day, you would be sure to find any combination of the Sibs and our daughters strolling up and down the neighborhood streets, with the Sibs happy to claim the two girls as their own to any friendly strangers. Nothing makes Matt or me prouder.

Leah discovers No. 1 Bowditch Road, with its yellow door and navy-blue exterior, exactly .2 miles, or six houses, from ours as the Sibs' next rental property somewhere between 2:00 a.m. and 4:00 a.m. while she is helping out with Kaia, who is now six weeks old. On occasion, Leah sleeps in Kaia's room with her. She claims that she loves it, and that Kaia sleeps more peacefully when she is in there, but we know it's to give us a break for a night. We doubt that Leah gets much sleep, but whatever her real rationale, it is a gift for us.

No 1. Bowditch, "1B," as the Sibs nicknamed their new rental, becomes home to the four of them for the foreseeable future. None of them can imagine missing substantial time with Havi, and Covid still prohibits any of them from returning to their in-office work, so they can each maintain their jobs from Boston.

1B has two bedrooms and an attic that the Sibs convert into an additional office. While I am not privy to all the juicy stuff that happens at their house, I like peering out of my window each evening and seeing the foursome walking up our street in time for dinner, laughing and animated about whatever has gone on that day. Jacob and Mike share a wall between their two office spaces. On workdays, Jacob sits at a portable desk in the sunroom and Mike sprawls on the couch in the adjacent living room, scrolling through legal briefs and depositions, with the two of them choreographing phone calls so as not to interrupt the other; meanwhile, Erin and Leah rotate between the kitchen and the attic office.

But what is best is walking up to their house on numerous days and peeking in the window at Erin at the kitchen table, busy with a Zoom call—and how she immediately goes offscreen for a moment as soon as she notices Havi or Kaia with me outside her front door. In an instant, the door opens and she is on the threshold smothering them with kisses. Then she darts back to the kitchen and returns to her Zoom call and runs the show again at her company. And as Leah works through her PhD, she rearranges all of her meetings to be available whenever we need and chooses her classes strategically so that the timing doesn't interfere with our communal meals or the girls' bedtime routines. I worry, at times, that Leah isn't prioritizing her own important work, but every time I raise the issue with her, she changes the subject.

At least once per week, Kaia has a sleepover at 1B. The Sibs call it the "sleep farm," and apparently process our requests in this way on their own group text chain:

> 1B, December 15, 2020, 2:30 p.m.
>
> Erin: Hi guys, we just had a reservation request come in for the sleep farm from one Kaia Goldstein. Are we open tonight? I'm not at the front desk right now to confirm the schedule.
>
> Leah: Lol. We do have a vacancy as Ms. Knell just checked out.
>
> Erin: How convenient! And are maintenance and housekeeping around for services tonight? Maintenance (Jacob) and housekeeping (Mike).
>
> Jacob: Shoot—it's the holidays—so sorry. But for a VIP, I'm available.

The morning reports after Kaia has a night at the sleep farm are generally positive, and funny too. The Sibs call Kaia "Lil Mama," and text us messages in the morning that make us laugh out loud: "Lil Mama did great. Slept from 7:30 p.m.–4:30 a.m. Aunt Leah did diaper change and Aunt Erin did bottle. Now snuggling in bed with J&E. Her visit with us can be extended through 9:00 a.m. if you like. We are almost out of breastmilk."

I don't fully understand how the four of them do it—navigate their professional lives, take care of themselves, and prioritize their own marriages, all while stepping in for Matt and me whenever we ask for help or they intuit we need support. I worry that the Sibs' devotion to us and to Havi and Kaia will take a toll on them. That they are delaying starting their own families, finding their own places to call home, and enjoying life as they should. I raise the issue with Jacob on a walk we take. "You know I'll more than understand when you need to get on with your life. Please. I want you all to be okay."

Without missing a beat, Jacob replies, "This is our life, Fra. Come on now."

We continue to talk openly about it—making sure they make time for their own "date" nights, even if that means missing dinner at our place and getting takeout from someplace else to eat at 1B; or going away for a weekend and spending time as a couple as opposed to a posse. But, over and over again, they choose Havi and Kaia. They never miss dinner, even though, occasionally, one of them needs to take a plate to go so they can return home to jump on a work call or finish a paper or prepare a presentation. For the most part, though, the six of us eat dinner together every single night, from the time the Sibs arrive in Boston in late spring until Havi's memorial service fifteen months later. We take turns having Havi and Kaia sit on our laps each night, and we pass Havi's smoothie cup from one set of hands to another, hoping that one of us will have better luck feeding her than the previous person. We rotate cooks and dishwashers, although Matt and Erin are most often the cooks, and the rest of us are on dishes. Jacob and Mike each have their own specialties too: for Jacob, it is grilled oysters, and for Mike, grilled peppers, zucchinis, and onions to top grilled veggie burgers.

* * *

According to the Sibs, the days unfold rather undramatically over at 1B, with everybody enjoying a cup of Jacob's morning brew and then each of them moving into their respective spaces for work. Erin texts everyone midmorning about a lunch order, and then by 5:00 p.m. they make the four-minute walk over to our house, all of them giving Havi and then Kaia as many kisses as possible as soon as they arrive. We eat ice cream every night after dinner, and I name myself "the scooper," taking great pride in knowing exactly what combination of scoops each of them wants. After ice cream, the Sibs all mosey back to 1B, where they often stay up late by the fire or watching *SportsCenter*. At bedtime, I am told, they establish a special call, "caw-cawwww," that one couple shouts to the other from their bedroom if the other's TV is too loud. I guess the cawing is much more polite than yelling, "Turn it down!"

Their close proximity is an amazing gift to us, and I know that adjusting to life without them is going to be hard, but that is a worry for another time.

* * *

We have an impossible conversation with Dr. Jo this week. The one when we began to talk about Havi's funeral, but we decide that we can't finish the conversation without Havi's input. It's not time for that just yet. Next up is her birthday, the last one we'll have with her here on this earth. How can that be?

CHAPTER 27

Turning Two

On Havi's second birthday, September 4, 2020, Matt and I whisk her away at midday to drive the familiar seven-and-a-half miles out to the suburb of Needham to Volante Farm, one of our favorite family-run farm stands. There, we spread her favorite pink-elephant blanket on the grass, unwrap the veggie sandwiches that we'd preordered, and eat lunch looking out across fields of kale, cucumbers, and squash. Havi takes her favorite snow-angel position on the blanket and closes her eyes. The sun is bright and warm, and the cloudless sky a perfect blue. Matt massages Havi's foot while I run my fingers through her hair. We both borrow her bib from time to time to wipe our faces as we devour our overstuffed avocado, cheese, and tomato sandwiches and finish lunch with two delicious ripe peaches. We make sure to dribble a few drops of peach juice onto Havi's lips.

Our conversation meanders between the mundane and the impossible, but whenever our minds drift too far from the pink elephant blanket, Havi brings Matt and me back to her and the here-and-now with a sigh or a coo. After lunch, we put her in the stroller and take a long walk around the beautiful Needham neighborhood. Granted, the celebration isn't the kind of birthday party that the average two-year-old dreams about, but we crossed into the world of Tay-Sachs, and there is no going back.

As Matt and I stroll, we talk about all the things that Havi has already been able to do in her short life. I turn to Matt, "she is already an older sister, a niece, a granddaughter, a cousin, and a friend. That's kind of amazing for someone who is only two years old."

No reply.

So I go on. "And you know she is the best listener and can silence a room with her giggle and turn heads with her mesmerizing beauty."

No reply. "Emmy?"

"Yeah, My, but she is also sick—the worst kind of sick, the kind of sick that can't go away over time or with rest or surgery or medication or cutting-edge treatment. And that's so fucked up. Why don't we get to rent a bouncy house and invite a dozen of her friends over? Why do we have to talk about her 'mesmerizing beauty'? She's two."

He's right and I agree, but I pick a fight instead. "Yeah, no shit Matt. But we don't have a bouncy house. So, get over it. This is her last birthday with us, is that how you want to be? I am so worried about you and I don't have the capacity to care for you too today." Matt just stares off in the distance, clearly hurt. I could see him pulling everything in.

That night, we collapse into bed and sleep hard, waking up the next morning to another beautiful 75-degree, blue-sky, full-sun September day. Looking out the bedroom window we see our backyard being transformed. Our families are there, prepping for Havi's birthday party that would somehow manifest all the fun of a great celebration as well as the mysticism of the incomprehensible. The party details are still a surprise to us, though our family makes sure that we are generally okay with the concept of gathering to celebrate Havi's birthday one last time.

By morning our backyard is transformed into a dining and dance hall ready for a party to begin at midday. Everyone makes sure that the party is Covid-safe by ordering individual boxed lunches for the fifty or so guests. Six picnic tables appear on the lawn, each featuring a bowl of blueberries and a flower arrangement as centerpieces and big mustard yellow balloons spelling out HAVI hangs from the stone wall that separates our yard from the protected land just behind our house, and several coolers are lined up in a row and filled with beers, wine, and seltzer.

Another of my college soccer teammates and best friends, Ali, with her husband Greg, travel from Geneva, New York. Ali and I played every minute of every college game together, never more than a few feet away from each other in the midfield. In big and small ways, she always had my back. As ever-present members of Havi's posse, they save her birthday decorations when Greg speeds off to a nearby Party City to collect a critical "A" balloon letter that floats away before the celebration begins.

In the space between our house and our neighbor's, and beneath a huge umbrella, a performance space is set up for the Hudson Project, a popular New York City-based events band that played at both my siblings' weddings. The Hudson Project's musical genre ranges from singer-song writer to soul, hip hop, and R&B. Andrea, the band's lead singer, is so touched by Jacob and Leah's reaching out to her to play at Havi's birthday party that the band makes a special, last-minute road trip up from New York City to sing and dance with Havi. In all of 2020, as Covid raged, Havi's birthday is the only gig the Hudson Project plays.

For the festivities, I dress Havi in a beautiful white and blue dress that enhances her angelic features. As our guests arrive, everyone greets her gently, often with a long, deep soulful stare. Soon after the party starts, as people eat and make chit-chat, Tia dances with Havi to reggaeton on our back patio. Later, Matt and I dance with Havi to "Landslide" and "Have I Told You Lately" in the middle of our backyard, as everyone else looks on, sways, and cries along with us. Andrea can't get through either song without crying herself.

Havi naps in her rocker on the patio, a faint smile on her sleeping face, her golden curls lit by the afternoon sun. The rest of us—Matt and me, Havi's aunts and uncles, grandparents, and close friends—sit in the backyard, weeping, as we watch a video of ourselves and other family and friends sharing their favorite moments with Havi during the two years of her life. No kids. No cake. No clown. No toys strewn about. No wishes on the candles. This is our toddler's birthday party.

When the video ends, so does the party, with a slow, tender, meditative rendition of the happy birthday song. We sing it in a circle, swaying together, our arms around each other's shoulders, commemorating Havi's last birthday on this earth.

When the last goodbyes are sobbed, I stand in the empty kitchen, holding her to my chest. As always when I hold Havi, her legs are wrapped around my waist. Gently, I tilt her head back. I look deeply into her eyes. "Was it okay today?" I ask my dying daughter. "Did you enjoy your party?"

Havi looks back at me solemnly for a long moment. Then she breaks out into the deepest, fullest giggling fit of her life.

In that moment, with Havi laughing in my arms, her beautiful eyes gazing straight into mine, a message comes to me. *Live with fullness*, it says. Surround yourself with people who matter. With music and dancing. With good food and bubbly drinks. With laughter and tears. Without pretense or façades. Devote yourself to what's most important. Hold nothing back. Live where boundless love and bottomless pain meet and mix.

CHAPTER 28

Blind

Simply the title of Jack Kornfield's book, *After the Ecstasy, the Laundry,* is enough to capture the liminal existence we lead with Havi, navigating between everyday life and our sacred time with her. Dr. Jo shares Kornfeld's work with us during a recent phone call and afterward, I read his most popular book that perceptively and incisively characterizes the stark and disorienting contrast we feel between our sacred moments with Havi and the more mundane moments of work, paying the bills, and cleaning the house.

Soon after Havi's birthday party, fall arrives. The days shorten noticeably and the light is different. When we step outside in the morning, the air is cool and crisp, the kind that makes you inhale reflexively and deeply, all the smells of summer's fading bloom. It is Havi's kind of weather, and we take her outside every day.

It is a time of endings, of letting go. Labor Day, Havi's birthday, and the end of my maternity leave all fall during the same week. After one particularly long day of Zoom meetings, Matt and I meet in Havi's bedroom as she wakes up from one of many naps in her little rocker. We pull up the window shade to let the dappled afternoon light dance across her legs and onto the rug, and in response she lifts her chin and rocks back and forth with small movements full of big love. I bend down and put my lips close to her ear and say, "I missed you today, sweetie," kissing her nose and cheek. She smiles and squeals and giggles; maybe she missed me that day, too. I doubt it. Then, as I pull back to gaze down at her, a tear runs down my nose and drops onto her leg; my lip quivers. I wish she knew how to miss me.

* * *

"I don't know if I should tell you this," Tia says one afternoon as Matt and I walk in from grocery shopping. We put down the bags we're carrying.

Tia sits at the table with Kaia and Havi, and she has tears in her eyes. "I don't think Havi can see us anymore," she says. "I think she's completely blind."

She nuzzles her face into Havi's hair and holds her close, whispering, "*Yo la amo*" in her ear, just as she has since the day they met. Tia, our ultimate optimist, our consummate source of joy and love, is looking crushed in a way I have never seen before and I don't know how to respond. The truth is, I have chosen not to explore the state of Havi's vision for months now. I made that decision the moment we finished the least helpful visit to the ophthalmologist back in December 2019, a week after Havi's diagnosis.

I know her whole face still changes when she hears Tia come through the front door in the morning. I know Havi sleeps better in Matt's lap than in our bed. I know she lights up when doted on by her aunts and uncles and grandparents. I know her chin lifts and her eyes brighten when I snuggle with her in the mornings. I know that when I hold her close and whisper in her ear, she turns toward me and looks deeply into my eyes and soul. I know that while Tay-Sachs is taking everything from her—her vision, movement, hearing, voice, laughter—it never touches our endless love for her. And there are no new baselines required to know any of that.

As fall comes on, our world is growing darker too, and our time feels even more precious. All we can do is continue to do everything we can to let Havi feel this world and to leave her fingerprints everywhere. In mid-September, we spend a weekend in New Hampshire's White Mountains, recharge back at home, and then the following weekend head back to Cape Cod to celebrate Havi's fortieth Shabbirthday and Rosh Hashanah.

Grandma and Grandpa, the Sibs, Kelsey and her boyfriend, and Tia and her husband make the trip with us. We want to give Havi and Kaia the High Holiday experience they deserve, and as we prepare to go, we do a lot of packing and unpacking: smoothies, rocker, onesies, bibs, medicines, pacifier, travel crib, sound machine, stroller, diapers, wipes. In the end, we have so much stuff that it looks like we're leaving for a month, not just a forty-eight-hour getaway.

In the car, sitting in the backseat as I always do between Havi and Kaia, I sometimes feel like I have whiplash. I look over at Kaia, and she smiles and sometimes screams; then I look over at Havi, and she seizes up, or has tremors, or sleeps. Then turn back to Kaia, who calmly sucks on a pacifier, and then to Havi, at her spasming legs and withering strength, and think again about how there is no remedy.

As soon as we arrive at our Airbnb on Cape Cod, Havi starts throwing up: in the car, the stroller, and finally on the living room rug while I change her clothes. It is scary, and even after such an immense emptying of her stomach, she is not interested in the bottle. She locks her lips, turns her head, and bites the straw so I can't even get one ounce into her. Then Tia happens to pour some of the same milk we use for Havi's smoothies into her own cup of coffee. "Um, oh, eh, ugh, this milk is very bad," she says. Matt opens the fridge and takes out the three glass jars of premade smoothies and he and I sniff them and nearly gag. "Very bad" is an understatement. Spoiled milk. All we can do is laugh.

Leah races out to get fresh milk, and Matt makes new smoothies. Havi is hesitant to sip it at first, and I don't blame her, but when she realizes the milk is okay, she sucks down nearly an entire bottle. It feels good to be able to solve a problem.

At our rental, Grandma spends two days preparing a delicious Rosh Hashanah dinner—not an easy task, ever, and that year she's up against our vegetarian, gluten-free, lactose-light diet. It is tough to do the traditional brisket veggie style. Plus, facing the reality of it being Havi's last Rosh Hashanah and Kaia's first, the words *"L'shana Tova"*—Happy New Year—are not exactly rolling off our tongues like they used to. But despite everything, dinner is delicious, and we savor every bite along with being together and still being with Hav.

Later that weekend, by Cape Cod Bay, we observe Tashlikh, a reflective Rosh Hashanah ritual traditionally performed near a body of water. Matt holds Havi in his arms and I hold Kaia in my chest carrier as I read aloud Malka Heifetz Tussman's poem, "Today is Forever," in Havi's honor. The poem speaks to my soul. It sings of streams and babbling creeks that flow endlessly; flitting butterflies and birds; flora that flourishes year-round: all turning and returning, as the High Holidays exhort us to do. Tussman concludes, "Today is forever. Forever is right now." I meditate on those words, wanting to believe them.

CHAPTER 29

Loss Before Loss

We grow increasingly worried about Havi. She sleeps more, eats less, and chokes often when she does try to ingest her smoothie, so we reluctantly reach out to the palliative care team we met with shortly after her diagnosis and set up a virtual appointment. We have two main objectives: (1) to understand what resources are available should we need additional support for Havi, especially at nighttime; and (2) find out what will happen if/when she develops a pneumonia or some other illness. Matt and I join the morning Zoom call on the morning of Havi's forty-first Shabbirthday, September 25, after we finish breakfast and put the girls down for naps.

The smiling face of the palliative care doctor stares back at us through the screen, looking phony, as if to say, "Here's my best attempt at looking empathetic like they said to do in the textbook, but clearly I have no idea how deep and dark and endless your pain is." Or maybe she was just afraid of our pain. I couldn't blame her for that. Our pain is terrifying. She hadn't been at our first in-person meeting back in February.

Midway through the Zoom call, I am in the middle of updating the doctor and her team on how Havi is doing when a little chat box pops up at the bottom of the screen: "She needs hospice," it reads. It is from the doctor. Immediately, on screen, she brings both hands to her mouth, looking horrified and embarrassed. I swallow hard and finish the sentence I am speaking at the time. She quickly and very professionally explains that she had just sent a chat message, one that was meant to be private—to another palliative care team member—to everyone on the call.

Seeing the word "hospice" in writing jolts Matt and me. We are not oblivious to Havi's needs—our care objectives for her have been and would continue to be what hospice tries to do: offer comfort at home. But our seeing that message is just another example of the medical system failing to provide the basic quality and humanity of care that we and Havi need. It is an especially difficult moment for Matt, who has worked so hard and so long to become a part of the medical system, which he views with such respect, even awe. He accomplished a decade of training only to realize how shockingly and horrifically broken the medical establishment is, and that the term "healthcare" is meaningless in a system that focuses on neither "health" nor "care." His words.

That night, Erin makes Havi a Shabbirthday blueberry cobbler that we use to double up the dose of deliciousness in Havi's smoothie, and she loves it, slurping down a whole bottle at dinner and taking in more ounces than she'd had all day. Maybe she has more time, after all, I dare to let myself think. At this point, I know we don't have years left with her. But I am hoping for many more months.

October arrives before we know it and with it comes Yom Kippur, the most holy day on the Jewish calendar, on Monday, October 3. Matt and I take the day off from work, but there is no fasting for us this Yom Kippur. The deep introspection that accompanies a twenty-four-hour fast doesn't feel necessary, so we decide to honor the holiday in a different way. We grab a blanket, toss Havi's stroller in the car, and head with her to World's End, a picturesque land preserve aside the Atlantic in Hingham, Massachusetts, about twenty miles south of our home. Kaia stays home with Tia. We pack a light lunch for another picnic: four slices of cold pizza, two dark-chocolate peanut butter cups, and two apples for Matt and me; and a world-class, homemade smoothie with extra blueberries and a scoop of Madagascar vanilla ice cream.

Our car ride is uneventful and feels short. When we arrive, we place Havi in the stroller and head for the carriage pathways that course along rolling hills and rocky shorelines. We intend to walk with her for a long while before eating, but the anticipation of cold pizza wins the day and we pretty quickly find a spot to sit and set up lunch. In front of us is Hingham Bay, with a view of the Boston skyline and beyond that the ocean; behind us are tree-lined trails with everchanging fall foliage. We spread out the pink-elephant blanket, and Matt lies Havi down so she can get a good look at the fall beauty around us. Matt and I each hold a pizza slice in one hand and Havi's tender hand in the other. She smiles as she tracks the afternoon light playing on the orange, red, and yellow leaves overhead and breathes in the blended scent of ocean air and red cedar trees.

And despite the place's rather ominous-sounding name, we soak up the boundless life pulsating all around us at World's End.

When Havi starts her *I'm hungry* grunting, I pick her up and place her on my lap so she can slurp down her smoothie as we look out at the water. She finishes with a satisfied burp. Suddenly, the sky is cloudy. Havi tips her head back and closes her eyes, and plop, a raindrop lands on her cheek. She scrunches up her nose. A second drop lands. Within ninety seconds, the sky opens up and it really starts to rain. Matt and I smile. Every time a raindrop lands on Havi's cheek, she scrunches up her nose, closes her eyes, and winces a little. She doesn't love it. We pack up quickly and huddle for a moment underneath a red autumn oak tree, thinking it might pass, but it doesn't, so we bundle Havi back into the stroller and high-tail it to the car. Matt and I laugh with her as she bounces along.

It is perfect—the best Yom Kippur we've ever had. Just as World's End's name belies all of the life there, so too, does Havi's mesmerizing beauty belie the ugliness of Tay-Sachs.

* * *

The hospice nurse speaks first. "When people hear the term hospice, they generally think of elderly people. We want you to know this is different. Pediatric hospice is different from traditional hospice." She opens her laptop as she sits across from Matt and me and another member of the palliative care team in our living room. Havi sits quietly on my lap.

Matt and I glance at each other, and then back at the nurse. She hasn't introduced herself, so we don't know her name. *Children aren't supposed to die.* Of course, pediatric hospice is different from regular hospice. We sit in uncomfortable silence. The social worker speaks next. "Your daughters both have such unusual names. Oh, and do you guys generally take your shoes off in the house? I notice you both have socks on."

I am not sure where to start. Matt is speechless. "Thanks," I say. I should have said, "They have *beautiful* names." *Unusual* stings. "And don't worry about your shoes," I add. Silence falls again.

There isn't much to talk about. We want to know who to call in case Havi gets really sick and we don't know what to do. So we have that phone number now. And we now know someone can be at our house within an hour.

Then, of course, there is paperwork. The nurse hands me a form to fill out. She explains that I am consenting to admitting Havi for hospice services. I write Havi's name first on the patient line. I mark X on the line that asks for patient signature. On the line requesting an explanation for why the patient can't sign, I simply write: *Age*. Then I sign my name as her legal representative. Matt signs his as Havi's witness.

More paperwork, more signatures, more reminders that we are signing Havi away. I had always assumed I'd sign for her until she was eighteen years old—tardiness to school, permission to go on field trips, a billion other things. *Pediatric hospice?* I don't even know how to process that. After a dispirited fifteen-minute visit, the nurse and the social worker leave. Matt and I pack up the girls and head out for ice cream.

Then Havi smiles her way through another week. *She can still smile.* What a gorgeous thing it is. It makes me realize we should all pay more attention to the power of a smile—to the strength and determination it takes to smile, to really smile.

* * *

October 10, 2020

Dear Peanut,

We had our appointment with Dr. Jo this morning. We are trying to prepare for the most horrible moment, the most difficult moment, the moment that marks the beginning of our endless grief. We cannot ever prepare or be prepared; we will only be able to check off the necessary logistics and ask our amazing people to help with things that we know we want, or don't want, or that we won't be able to manage when that day arrives.

I'm not doing well with any of it. I guess that's expected. The thing is, we are okay right now, in these present moments, because we have you with us physically. You are here: We scoop you up every morning; we place you in between us and snuggle you up in our bed; we hold you for all your meals; we dance with you; we kiss you a thousand times every day; and we tuck you in and sing you to sleep every night. And even as you lose everything, having your warm body curled up in our arms makes it possible to get through a day. And the thing is, in what I call "the long long," I know, or at least I hope, we'll be okay even when we don't have you physically. I see amazing people like Charlie and Blyth and Dr. Jo, whose lives are rich, beautiful, filled with love, and full of pain, and they all seem okay. But Havi girl, what lies in between these two, in between the present and the long long, is dark, painful, and uncertain, and that scares me. Because the truth is, losing you will never be okay.

You've had a remarkably good week and I've felt so close to you these past few days. Maybe it's the chill of the fall air but you seem to be snuggling even closer. You, me, Kaia, and Mom were sitting on the couch last night before dinner. I had you tucked in my left arm, your legs stretched across my lap, and your head resting against my shoulder and turned slightly up toward mine. Your face was close, I could hear your little breaths and smell your skin. I looked down and your big beautiful brown eyes were fixed on mine. You held them there for long minutes that I lost track of. You put a lifetime's worth of conversations into that gaze, sweet girl. After we put you to bed I started to tell your mom about that moment. Before I could finish my sentence, she said, "I saw it too. I saw it too."

We love you.

Dad

* * *

At 9:15 p.m. one Monday in mid-October, Matt and I lie in bed staring at the ceiling. "I miss her," I whisper and turn over to face Matt.

"I do, too. I always miss her. And she's not even gone yet," Matt says.

Havi has been asleep for nearly two hours, and while there is nothing particularly unique about this night, except that the date, October 12, signifies that time is moving quickly, and I want time to stop.

"I am going to get her. She can snuggle with us for a bit tonight," I leap out of bed and creep into Havi's dark, cozy room to kidnap her. I scoop her up from her rocker, carry her into our bedroom, and lay her gently down on my pillow. Our lights are on. She opens her eyes wide, as if she is ready for a new day.

"Emmy, she looks wide awake!" I say to Matt, and he looks over at me as if to say, *Of course she's wide awake. You woke her up in the middle of a deep sleep and brought her into our fully illuminated room.*

But he just smiles, and says, "I'm kind of glad she's up."

Then Havi unleashes a huge smile and stretches out as best she can. She moves her head gently from side to side, and Matt and I sandwich her with our bodies. I turn the lights off. *This is actually quite nice; we should do this more*, I think to myself while dozing off to sleep.

Moments later, though, I hear Havi's disgruntled mumble, and worry that our magical moment has passed. But soon her breathing turns to snoring. "It's not safe to let her lie on her back," I ruin the moment.

"I know Love, but she is okay. We are right here. Let's let her sleep for a few minutes."

She startles awake only moments later, and our sleepover ends abruptly. Matt lifts her out of bed and holds her tightly as he carries her across the hall to her rocker. I follow him and then we tuck her in for the second time. She lets out a gentle sigh; we kiss her cheeks and forehead and leave her room for the night. "See you in the morning," we say together—parting words that we hold onto tightly. Matt pauses before closing the door, "Goodnight sweet girl, I love you."

We get back into bed. "Can you snuggle me from behind tonight? I need to feel you close," Matt says to me.

"Yeah, I'm here. Right here," I say as I wrap my arm around his waist.

And then it is morning, and our routine of medicine and breakfast smoothies begins anew. We are in a daily rhythm with Havi and Kaia of work, intermittent cuddles, seizures, diaper changes, spit-up, smoothie slurping, and neighborhood walks.

It is hard to see Havi's fragile and failing body draped over Tia's shoulder or passed from one set of arms to another without any of her own strength to guide her, or the glazed-over look that is more and more filling her mesmerizing eyes. I hate that she is confined to a Fisher Price rocker chair with a polyester seat cushion that vibrates for twenty minutes and then shuts off, and that she's developed a rash between her thumbs and her index fingers on both hands because she can no longer move them. Her little hands are raw and red and look so painful and, like everything else, they will never heal. And when she's drooling and her eyes are at half-closed, I hate that it's hard for me to look at her. I feel pathetic.

And on the days when it all becomes too much, Matt and I sneak out for a neighborhood run or walk, to either talk or not talk.

On this walk, we talk about the future, the present, and the past, meandering through memories and fears. I describe to Matt a moment that Havi and I shared the previous summer when we were at the Cape and I carried her down near the water. She and I stood beneath a cluster of towering trees. She wrapped her legs around my waist and I placed her arms up on my shoulders and whispered in her ear, "You're going to get a second chance. You must." And then she squeezed her legs around my waist, as if to say, *I know, Mom.*

Matt stops in his tracks. "Why does she have to have a second chance? Who is she going to be with? Why can't she just be with us? Why can't she just have her first chance with us?" All of a sudden it becomes hard for me to breathe. I said the wrong thing. Matt cries through a series of impossible questions for which I have no answers. He walks ahead of me. "Can you please come back?"

"I need a minute. I'll meet you at home."

We round the cul-de-sac and head for home. Matt is a few yards ahead of me. I want to catch up, but I know I shouldn't. So I stay behind. Are we going to be okay? I wonder to myself as I kick a rock and follow its path.

* * *

Matt takes a shower before Shabbirthday dinner. Later that night, he writes his journal entry with Havi on his lap.

October 24, 2020

Hi Havi,

I had one soapy arm and an empty bottle of body wash in my hand. The hot water hit my head, shoulders, and chest and ran in streams down to the drain. I tried, for a moment, to spread the suds around but I was too sweaty and funky for a soapless water rinse. So I reached my arm out of the shower and put the empty bottle on the counter as a reminder to get new soap. And then I turned back to the shelf in the corner and moved around the bottles. An old bottle of your baby soap was propped against the wall in the back, tipped upside down and balanced just so to get the little remaining bit down to the opening. It was the bottle we had taken with us on the Havimoon, back in January. I remember pulling it out of the suitcase when we got back to Boston so I could give you a shower after that long travel day. We showered with you a lot during that time out on the California coast. And in beautiful hotel showers with big fluffy, white towels that Mom would wrap you up in as soon as you were all clean.

I looked at that little bottle and took a deep breath. It has been months since I showered with you. We've fallen back into our pre-Havimoon routine and have been bathing you in the bathtub in that little pink bath seat that we used in the first days after we brought you home from the hospital and being born. You're much too big for it now, you know. But it's the only way to make the bath work. Your head reaches the top edge and your arms and legs spill over the sides and dangle in the water. You look almost intentional in your lounging. And you rock your head side-to-side as we pour warm water gently over your chest and belly, your legs and feet, and down the back and sides of your neck. And when our knees start to hurt from the tile floor, we flip the drain and say goodbye to the bath water. And when I lift your wet body up, your arms and legs hang limply behind you and your head falls back, leaving your beautiful neck stretched and exposed. There is nothing intentional in this.

How is it that your beautiful body can be failing you so badly?

Later on today, I bought the biggest bottle of your baby soap I could find and put it in the middle of the shower shelf. And now every morning I can smell you in soap and feel you hanging over my shoulder, spinning slowly in a circle letting the water run over and around us together.

Physics teaches us that energy can neither be created nor destroyed; rather; it can only be transformed or transferred from one form to another. What will you be when you leave us, sweet girl?

We love you.

Dad

*   *   *

The next night, Charlie and Blyth come over for dinner. I sit inside with Blyth, and Matt and Charlie stay by the firepit on the deck off our kitchen. I tell Blyth I think Havi is getting more distant, harder to reach. Sometimes I feel like I don't even know her. Or that she doesn't even know me. "She's cocooning, turning inward," Blyth responds and puts her hand on my leg. She continues. "She's no less herself, I promise. Just not sharing as much. Our therapist recommended we read Trina Paulus's book *Hope for the Flowers* when Cameron was at this stage. It helped."

Turning inward. This makes sense. Blyth always knows what to say. Sitting across from Blyth, I am in awe of her strength and her capacity to guide me in the least patronizing and most reassuring way.

"You seem untouchable to me, Blyth."

"Cameron is my kryptonite," she replies and picks up each of our plates, bringing them to the sink.

On the following morning, I open the front door to bring the garbage cans up from the street. A bag is on the doorstep. There's a book inside. It's *Hope for the Flowers*. Matt and I sit in the living room and read it in one sitting. We cry as we read these lines:

Watch me. I'm making a cocoon.

It looks like I'm hiding, I know, but a cocoon is no escape.
It's an in-between house where the change takes place.
It's a big step since you can never return to caterpillar life.
During the change, it will seem to you or to anyone who might peek that nothing is happening—but the butterfly is already becoming.
And, there's something else!
Once you are a butterfly, you can really love—the kind of love that makes new life. It's better than all the hugging caterpillars can do.

CHAPTER 30

To Kaia from Havi

October 31, 2020

Dear Kaia,

It's me, Havi. Mom is writing for me. I want to share this with you so you can hear my voice and read this one day when things are different. People may ask you about me, and you may have lots of questions yourself, so I want you to have something directly from me. Maybe it'll give you comfort or guidance, or maybe it'll just be a way to imagine the sound of my voice when I'm gone.

You are four months old today. It feels like not so long ago that Mom and Dad left for the hospital and I stayed home with Aunt Leah and Grandi, waiting for your arrival. I was excited and nervous. I watched you grow in Mom's belly and I wondered what you would be like. I wanted everything to be just right when you got home. We made you a sign that we hung from our kitchen window that we didn't take down for weeks! It said: WELCOME HOME, KAIA LEV!

It was an instant love affair between the two of us. You were so tiny, with lots of dark hair on your head. And you slept a lot so I got to tuck you under my arm and hold you close. We snuggled on the moon-pod beanbag in the corner of the kitchen and sat together on Mom's lap in the rocking chair in your room; we snoozed together on Dad's chest on the couch downstairs and napped side by side in my room. We took long walks together around the neighborhood. You let me lie next to you on your playmat and you even let me snuggle up to you in your boppy pillow that Mom and Dad place at the center of the kitchen table. You are loving and playful with me, even though I can't reciprocate in the way I always imagined I would.

We went to the beach together on Cape Cod and we explored New Hampshire. We celebrated my second birthday and the Jewish Holidays. But we've spent most of our time together in our home in Boston. Make sure you ask Mom and Dad about how much we laughed and smiled together. They're taking so many pictures all the time, sometimes it's annoying, but I know that those pictures will be nice for you to have later on. You wear a lot of my old clothes (and your cousins Ayla's and Hannah's old clothes). I love knowing that we share pajamas. Maybe our dreams get passed to each other through them. I think my favorite part about you is that you smile with your whole body. I can see your smile even when you're turned away from me because your face changes shape and you crunch up your arms and your legs into a full body smile.

Our bedtimes are synced now. Sometimes you join Mom and Dad for my bedtime routine. They say goodnight to the bay every night and sing "Have I Told You Lately" and "Wonderful Tonight" with me. And I love that you join in now. I've heard Dad singing "Stand by Me" to you at night. It sounds like you now have your bedtime song, too. Our rooms share a wall, and I like knowing that you're just on the other side. I can hear you sigh in your sleep sometimes, and I want you to know that I'm never far away.

Now, this is the not-so-fun part. I won't get to watch you grow up. And we won't get to grow up together. There is so much I want to tell you, Kai—so much about our parents, our aunts and uncles and grandparents, and all the amazing friends who love us so much—but I can't. It's true what you'll read about Tay-Sachs. It's a cruel and devastating disease and it took a lot away from the two of us, and from our family. And it will take everything away from me. It's also true that there is a very long list of all the things I never did, that we never did together, some of the simplest things, the things that most of us take for granted: move, see, talk, eat, even go to the bathroom on your own! So, to the extent that you can, do those things! And maybe through you, I'll get to feel and experience them too.

I can't wait for you to take your first steps, or for you to say hi to Mom and Dad. They've been waiting a long time to hear those words. I probably won't be physically with you for most of these moments. I'm really sad about that. But I'm not writing to you so that you worry about me. I'm writing to you so you know how much I love you.

I want you to live a beautiful life. When you can't see me, or when the world seems to be moving fast and you've got lots going on, maybe you'll feel me. At some point, you'll know I'm right there with you doing all the things together.

The thing about sisters is that there's a whole lot of unbreakable energy between them. And we're no different. So when anyone asks, "Are you the oldest?" the answer should always be, "NO! I have an older sister!" But I'd also understand if sometimes it's easier, less confusing for people, for you, to answer however you want. Because I'll know exactly what you mean, and I'll never take offense. I promise you that.

I'd tell you to take care of Mom and Dad but they are solid and that's not your job. So just laugh with them a lot. They are good at that. And here are the high points on them: They operate as a team, they love us a lot, and if anything ever gets tense, make sure they go out for a long run, preferably together.

Just be a kid. I never got the chance to do that, and it seems like a lot of fun. Look around a lot, too. Don't spend too much time in your own head, you might miss a gust of wind, a purple leaf, or a beautiful sunset trying to tell you what matters. The world is big, so squeeze everything you can out of it, for we don't know how much time we have in this beautiful place with all of our beautiful people.

We had a busy week and we're all feeling ready for the weekend. We celebrated my forty-sixth Shabbirthday last night during our first snowfall of the season. I'm already so proud of you, and I always will be. And when this letter doesn't feel like enough, I'm feeling the same way. Never be afraid to talk about me, to ask about me, to ask about all the adventures Mom, Dad, and I had. I want you to know all of me.

I love you, Kaia.

Your big sister,

Havi

CHAPTER 31

Pneumonia

On the morning of November 4, we wake up to Kaia's usual staccato yell that closely approximates the sound of two cats fighting. It is 4:45 a.m. and Matt and I pull ourselves out of bed bleary-eyed from having stayed up late to watch Donald Trump and Joe Biden election night coverage on CNN. We'd finally gone to bed feeling a bit out of sorts with nothing having been decided yet.

Around 7:00 a.m., Matt and I peek in Havi's room. Usually she is stirring by now, but this morning her eyes are closed, she snores a little, and she looks so peaceful that we decide to wait to scoop her up. But then it is 7:15, 7:30, 7:45, and she still hasn't stirred. Finally, at 8:00, we wake her. The front of her pajamas is soaked from saliva and she sounds congested as she breathes. When we lay her gently on the changing table, she starts to cough hard, and when we sit her up, she vomits. "Em, I'm scared. Is this it?" I get Havi's arm stuck in her pajamas as I try to take them off. "Breathe, My. No. I don't think so. But let's get her out of these wet pajamas."

We change her into fresh clothes and carry her to the kitchen for breakfast. She slurps down a few ounces of morning smoothie, but it isn't much compared to what she'd been having during meals over the last few weeks. I am counting ounces now. Something Charlie said he used to obsess over, too. By midday her cheeks are flushed, and she is hot to the touch. We take her temperature—102.7 F— and get a few doses of infant Tylenol into her mouth with a syringe; by dinnertime she perks up a bit and her fever is down. She drinks a few more ounces of smoothie on my lap at the dinner table and falls asleep. We bring her to her rocker, and make a plan to check on her every few hours through the night. Matt and I alternate shifts, and each time, she feels cool. We don't sleep much, and neither does Kaia—we get the feeling that she too knows something is up with Havi.

The next morning Havi doesn't have a fever when we wake her, but she is still lethargic and groggy. When we bring her to the kitchen, she drinks a few ounces of smoothie, slowly. Maybe it takes her five minutes per ounce. By midmorning her fever is back: 103.6 F. It has to be pneumonia. Blyth and Charlie warned us of this. Pneumonia can kill children with Tay-Sachs. Havi lies limply in my arms and I can't get her to drink anything. I try the bottle in her mouth a dozen times before giving up. My chest is tight. Matt makes a flurry of phone calls, to the Sibs and to the hospice team, and a nurse is scheduled to come to our house with a dose of antibiotics. Next comes a medication delivery—morphine, Ativan, and Tylenol suppositories, all of which we store in the fridge next to a block of cheese—followed by an emergency medical equipment truck, bringing us an oxygen machine just in case we need it. Ironically, this overly large machine is delivered by a very small man. Erin tucks the machine deep into the back of Havi's closet after getting a brief tutorial.

Then the nurse arrives. Havi sits on my lap on the living room couch with her eyes closed and I hold her hand. The needle is big. I am afraid of needles. I look away, but hold her close. She barely makes a sound as the antibiotics are injected into her thigh. As we spin into night two of whatever this is, my thoughts go to the darkest places. *Are we in our last weeks or days with Havi?* I am not ready. I panic. I want more time, more memories, more kisses, more goodnight lullabies, even more medicine-infused smoothies. I don't really care what our days look like—I just want more of them. I feel desperate. Matt appears steady.

Aunt Leah and Aunt Erin stay overnight to help. The four of us take turns sneaking into Havi's room to kiss her head, rub her legs, and wake her up every four hours for another rectal Tylenol suppository and another attempt at drinking a few ounces of smoothie. As the night wears on, she seems steadily better. At 1:00 a.m., I even catch Havi's aunts giggling with her. Pneumonia in our house doesn't have to mean no laughter. Leah recounts the night to us the next morning: "We fumbled our way in the dark—making several clumsy attempts and wasting suppositories, doing multiple thermometer-reads and made panicked Celsius to Fahrenheit conversions, with a pair of glasses flying across the room in frustration at one point. Hav seemed totally calm, though, and even gave us the courtesy of a few sacred giggles, patiently waiting for us to get our act together."

* * *

Friday morning brings us all a sense of relief: Havi is drinking again, her color is back, she smiles at me. Matt and I sit at the kitchen table, exhausted and preoccupied with a constant stream of worries. *Is her fever really gone? Is she in pain? Can we get another ounce of smoothie into her?* "Please, Havi girl," I always plead with her, "just a few more sips."

We are scared. What does her pneumonia mean? How long would it be until her next bout? Would there even be a next bout?

In this deepest fear, Matt and I fall more in love with Havi and appreciate how strongly we are programmed, as parents, to be cellularly connected to her. "I should bring her up to nap, now, Emmy."

"I'll come too."

We plant dozens of kisses on her cheek before we leave her room. And then let her nap.

* * *

Developmental delays. Missed milestones. Loss of strength. Inability to sit up. Difficulty swallowing. The end of solid food. Babbling replaced by coos and grunts. Loss of vision. Loss of laughter. Loss of smiling. Seizures. Pneumonia.

We have nearly run the course of everything Tay-Sachs would do to and take from her, except for the worst thing, the last thing. Matt and I acknowledge that we are in a new phase now, the last phase. There will be a few more battles ahead, and then it will be over. But we are not ready to say goodbye, and neither, we feel, is she. We will keep listening closely; she'll tell us when she needs to go.

But that bout of pneumonia takes it out of all of us. Especially Matt and me. The dark lines under our eyes made the Sibs worry and they take Kaia for a few sleepovers this week. In fact, Kaia gets to have nights with all three of her aunts: Aunt Leah, Aunt Erin, and Aunt Maggie, who has flown in again from Colorado. Our house is so quiet without Kaia. I walk by her empty room next to Havi's and catch my breath. Then I reassure myself: Kaia is only just down the street. We will see her the next morning, or even sooner if she gets upset and needs to come home.

Then my thoughts drift to Havi. When she recovers from her pneumonia, we find that she has lost even more of herself. It is harder for her to drink from a straw, so we transition to a simpler bottle with a plunger that allows us to control the flow. Eventually her bedroom will be empty too, with no return date for her. Thinking about that makes my chest tighten and my legs heavy. I quietly open her door and tiptoe up to her little sleeping rocker, being careful to avoid stepping on the floorboard that creaks, and sit on the floor on my knees next to her so I can breathe her scent in deeply. Then I give her a kiss on her forehead and creep back out of the room to walk downstairs, open the freezer, and scoop some ice cream into a bowl. The quiet makes me feel lonely in a way that scares me. I write a weekly journal entry to Havi about it:

> I dread the day when I'll sit down to write to you and I can't reach out to squeeze your hand, run my fingers through your hair, massage your little calves, or plant a big kiss on your red lips. And while it's true that your energy and your spirit have already transcended your physical being, there is so much of you encased in your gorgeous body. Trying to make sense of life without you, you who we brought into the world only two years ago, feels like emotional amputation.
>
> But today, I write with you here. And even though as I write you startle or choke or stiffen, I feel you and pick you up in my arms and hold you close when I need to be recentered. You shouldn't have to play that role, but you've become that person for me. The person I look to when I want to see the best in others or when I need perspective or patience, or purpose. And I'm scared of who I might become when we lose you. When you're out of reach. I can only hope that I'll find the softness and strength you bring with you everywhere you go; the way you, without uttering a word, say so much about what is important and what is not; the way you, without ever taking a single step, have

your footprints all over our incredible community and this beautiful Earth.

I am sitting with Havi in her rocking chair as we inch up toward the anniversary of Diagnosis Day, December 17. I gaze out her bedroom window at the gray sky and the cold air. My mind wanders around the moments of "this time last year" when we were so fucking hopeful, blind to the possibility of such devastation. I rub my lips against Havi's chin, and I can't stop shaking my head. And then I sink into the chair, readjust Hav's head against my chest, and sob.

CHAPTER 32

Pay Attention

Sometime that fall, on an impulse, we buy ourselves a firepit. It is the last one Home Depot has and unfortunately it is emblazoned with the New England Patriots logo. Despite living in Boston for almost ten years, I still am a devoted Philadelphia sports fan. We set the firepit up on the deck, just outside the kitchen, on a few gray stones to insulate the wooden planks from the heat. We spend a lot of fall and early winter nights sitting around it with the Sibs and my parents. In November, the burning wood smells rich and warm and the sleepy heat feels especially good against the cold.

Tonight, we sit out there when it is finally announced that Joe Biden has won the presidential election. On a laptop, we watch with the Sibs around the fire, his and Kamala Harris's speeches as a brisk wind swirls around us. I am brought back to the many cold mornings we sat with Havi in Tomales Bay by the fire when the water was still and the sky was misty. Matt and I would snuggle up with Havi and look out at the bay and whisper in her ear, "I love you, I've got you, I love you, I've got you."

Dr. Jo tells us that grieving over losing Havi will be excruciating, that it will be like sitting around one of these fires on a cold night. She compares the power of grief to the power of fire: It can consume us and devastate us, and it can also provide warmth and resonating light in the midst of the darkness that will fall upon us.

In some ways, these weeks while Havi recovers from pneumonia feel like stolen time. It has shaken me to my core and even felt, at times, like we have come right up against the moment I fear the most. But now, we find ourselves in a liminal space, an in-between space, where we don't fully belong to the world of the living or the world of the dead. We are at the edge of both, and our world is different from everyone else's. It feels like a holy space, not in a religious sense per se, but as if someone is grabbing me by the shoulder, shaking me, and demanding, "PAY ATTENTION!"

* * *

Thanksgiving 2020 starts with a morning rainfall. We construct a turkey trot to get us out in the elements. The adult girls run. Jacob pushes our two sleeping girls in a stroller up a steep hill. Matt makes sourdough bread at home. The day unfolds slowly. Erin and Kelsey cook. The boys toss a football outside. I sit holding Havi's face between my two hands and study her peaceful facial features—her mouth open, nostrils gently flared, eyeballs dancing beneath her eye lids; and I notice as her chest rises and falls against mine as she sleeps. I let the weight of her twenty-three-pound body ground me in this moment. I never sat for this long or appreciated the power of a quiet moment until Havi's diagnosis. I like this version of myself and I want to unmeet her if it means Havi is healthy.

Our family sits down for Thanksgiving dinner with a bigness in our hearts that feels palpable. The foods on our table feature nearly every color on earth: green beans and cranberry sauce and stuffing and delicata squash. Matt proposes a toast to Havi and we all raise our glasses as he remarks on both the joys and sorrows of this particular Thanksgiving, how holidays spur us into mental time-travel from the beauty and nostalgia of the past to the terror and loneliness that loom in our future.

We place Kaia, as our centerpiece, in her boppy lounger, right on the table, smack in the center of the action, so she can turn her head from side to side to take everything in, and we can bask in her cuteness. We strap Havi's rocker onto a wooden bench so she can join us at the table—we want her at eye level, right between Matt and me. She starts dinner in my lap with a first course of anti-seizure medicine administered by syringe—three milliliters worth, trickled into the corners of her mouth so she doesn't cough. She patiently swallows it all, and then drinks her smoothie as I keep her tucked under my arm. Midway through dinner, I pass her over our makeshift chair to Matt's lap. She nestles into her favorite spot. We make our way through second and third helpings and then take a break before dessert. Our laughter, storytelling, and overeating remind us of Thanksgivings past, and each forkful of stuffing, cranberry sauce, and blistered string beans make me feel normal, for just a moment. We never end up putting Havi into her rocker on the bench. She stays in our arms for all of dinner, where she belongs.

Matt speaks about how our feelings of grief and gratitude are hopelessly intertwined. I never appreciated how connected the two are with each other. We all hold hands, fingers crossed and wrapped in gentle firmness. We have so much to be grateful for, and so much to grieve. And I am bursting with all of it, the bright and the dark.

CHAPTER 33

Painful Anniversary

Havi is sleeping in more. Her typical 7 a.m. wake-up drifts toward 8 a.m. I understand why: She is tired and medicated, and who wouldn't want to stay snuggled beneath warm blankets on colder, dark mornings? In the pall of the morning after her fifty-second Shabbirthday, on December 12, I sit with Kaia and write to Havi:

> Dear Beauty,
>
> Kaia is to my right, playing with her feet and putting them (and everything she can get her hands on) in her mouth. She's quite chatty, too, and sweet, and self-satisfied. Some moments I catch a glimpse of you in her. But at other moments, it's hard to imagine that you were once as playful and bright as she. But you were! As I write I wonder whether it might sound to you like I'm comparing the two of you. I am not. I am only considering the ways in which you show up in her, the ways you are there for each other, and the ways I want to remember the two of you being contented by each other's side.
>
> Kaia's taken a particular interest in you lately. She reaches out for you, stares deeply at your perfect, porcelain skin and big, beautiful eyes, and strokes (okay, sometimes grabs) your curly blonde hair. I can almost hear her saying, "I love you. I admire you. I want to be near you." And sometimes she lets out a particularly deafening screech and you startle, but most times the two of you seem so in sync. It's impossible for me to imagine one of you without the other. And when I try, I'm overcome with pain.
>
> I imagine sometimes that what's happening must be confusing for you. There is a lot of love and pain wrapped

up in most moments of every day. And there are many times in a day when someone who loves you a lot looks deeply into your face with their eyes full of tears. So I want to be clear: We are loving more because of you. And we are hurting more because of Tay-Sachs. You are everything that is beautiful and nothing painful. You are the easiest person to love, and we've created the most magical love bubble for you, filled with our people, who know how to hold you so your head doesn't droop and how to support your spine in a way that sits you up into normal posture, who lean in and whisper, "I love you" in your ear in the midst of a seizure. When your dad and I watch other people with you, we sometimes can, for a brief moment, forget that you are sick.

More recently, Dad and I have been so struck by your patience and calm. We've been a little frenetic, trying to squeeze everything into your short life. But every day, you pull us back from the chaos of phones and calendars and deadlines. We dance with you more, we sing with you more, we stretch out our meals with you more. Maybe it is you yourself who is at the heart of the art of stillness.

We love you.

Mom

*   *   *

On December 17, 2020, the anniversary of Diagnosis Day, we awake to snow like last year when it lightly dusted the woods behind our house and in stark contrast we learned that Havi is dying in front of us. Today, the sky is dark gray and filled with thousands of little snowflakes that ride the wind back and forth across the window of our bedroom. The roof on the neighbor's house is smooth and white with neatly manicured corners and edges, as if someone has laid down a perfect layer of vanilla frosting across it. The world gets quiet when it snows, and Matt and I are glad, because we need some quiet today.

Our morning is slow and peaceful. Kaia is napping in her room. Matt and I start the day by cuddling Havi in the living room with the lights

157

turned low as we watch the snow pile up outside and wait for the plows to come up the street. As we feed her on the couch and she dozes off, the sky starts to lighten a little. We sit quietly with her for a while, watching her sleep, listening to her breathing and sneaking gentle kisses on her cheeks and forehead. We don't talk.

Once Kaia wakes up from her morning nap, Matt changes her diaper. Moments later, he walks into our bedroom with Kaia over his shoulder and a confused look on his face. "Kaia's not moving her right arm the way she used to. Seems fussy too."

"What do you mean?" I say, my voice panicked.

He lies her on our bed to show me. "I don't know what's going on." Matt says.

"Why are you being so vague? What do you mean you don't know?" I ask urgently. Developmental regression plays on repeat in my mind. I don't give him time to respond. "Are you worried?" My voice quivers.

"No, I don't think so. I mean, it could be something musculoskeletal. Let me call Dr. Laster. Maybe she will do a video call so she can see Kaia."

I stay with Havi in bed. How is this happening? I am spinning. *What the fuck is "musculoskeletal" and why can't he just use normal words?* Matt walks back into our room with a smile on his face and Kaia is babbling in his arms.

He says with lightness in his voice, "Before I could even finish the first sentence, Dr. Laster says: 'Nurse Maid's Elbow, named for nurses who, in a rush, would grab the babies in their care by the wrist or hand. Today, that type of injury is more often caused by fathers...!'"

I am not amused. "So, is she okay?"

"Yes, she's fine now. Dr. Laster gave me a few guiding instructions, I dusted off some old med school textbook pages, and reset her dislocated elbow. So, there it is, I dislocated and relocated Kaia's elbow all in the same morning."

"Please don't do that again," I snap angrily. I can't handle anything else.

I want laughter to come easily. But it doesn't. And I don't want to live in such generalized fear.

* * *

We all curl up on the couch downstairs. Matt turns on the video that the Sibs made for Havi's second birthday party and we watch, through streams of tears, some of the vibrant moments from Havi's much too short life. I hadn't heard Havi's giggle in a long time and the sound of it catches me and reverberates through my chest. We watch her feeding herself challah. We watch her stand. We watch her open her mouth widely into the biggest smiles, taking full bites out of her days. Matt and I cry. Kaia stares at the screen intently. I start to laugh when I remember that Charlie and Blyth told us that when Eliza was very young, she used to fake cry when they'd watch Cameron's birthday video to be a part of it.

That afternoon, Kaia practices crawling with her aunts in the living room. I hear the cheering and chanting from upstairs as Matt and I prepare to shower with Havi. I love that Kaia is starting to crawl. She is so ready. "Water's ready, My." I step into the bathroom. Matt is already in the shower with Havi, who tips her head back into his arms and lets the water run through her hair. As her golden curls turn dark and heavy with water, they reach almost midway down her back. When did her hair get so long? I wonder aloud. Then I join them. "I'm freezing, Emmy. Can I get under?" Matt laughs. Showering with him is one of my favorite things and we always end up laughing as I slowly crowd him out of the water. The day ends with a pizza delivery, and we sit with the Sibs on the couch, watching more Havi videos.

* * *

With the days growing colder and shorter, our lives become simpler in many ways. There are no big trips to think about or plan, no daily commutes to navigate, no appointments or meetings or dinner parties to attend. Our days are filled with home, with our daily routine nearly identical from one day to the next, and somehow, even in their monotony, the days feel like some of the most exhilarating times of our lives.

It is this sense of simplicity that I know I'll long for when Havi dies. It's a beautiful and rare thing to want to be exactly where you are, with no yearning for anything more or different, and instead, only a deep appreciation for what is, and who is right beside us. Being, not doing, takes practice. And for me, it takes my dying daughter to understand its power.

During these happy winter days, we experience a lot. We successfully manage to remove a stinkbug who sets up camp in our cozy, warm kitchen. When the weather suddenly turns warm, Matt and I wear shorts on back-to-back runs as the warmth wipes away the two feet of snow that had painted our world white. Havi and Kaia hold hands every morning. Kaia stands next to Havi's rocker and reaches for Havi, tugging on her pajama arms. Havi and Matt watch Christmas Day basketball, and she lifts her hand onto his while the two of them snuggle together on the couch. We celebrate Havi's fifty-fourth Shabbirthday over Chinese food with Grandi and Grandadders and eat so much that our bellies are still full nearly twelve hours later. And we raise a glass to Havi at that meal. Always to Havi.

As I pay close attention to all the beautiful nothings, there are moments when Havi feels so present and others when she feels really far away. Both scare me. When we feel connected, really connected, I can't in all of my imagination fathom life without her physical being. Thinking about it, I lose my breath, my chest tightens, my legs feel heavy and my eyes well up with tears. Then, in the moments when she feels so far away, like we've already lost so much of her, my sadness cascades into anger, fear, and loneliness and it all sits lodged like a golf ball in my throat.

My thoughts drift constantly to the childhood Havi will never have, to my own fears and insecurities as a mother, and to Kaia, her little sister, who has so much beautiful life ahead of her. My thinking goes something like: *We have new neighbors. They have healthy children. Havi should be playing with them. She never will. Havi is our first daughter. She is so beautiful, and so sick. She's never spoken a single word. She never will. I am Havi's mother. I am so scared and sad. But every day with her is a gift. Kaia seems healthy. But we're creeping up on the developmental milestones. Will she slip, too? Seems impossible to think she could. But Havi did.*

CHAPTER 34

The New Year

"Good riddance!" reads the headline on the *New York Times* the morning of January 1, 2021. The year 2020 was a hard one for everyone. Intellectually, I understand the sentiment of wanting to move past 2020. But for us, it is different. I want to hang onto 2020 forever, playing it on repeat like a favorite song. For us, 2020 stripped a lot away and laid bare the essence that is life. If it were another time, if Havi were healthy and normal, maybe 2020 would have been difficult, uncomfortable, scary: routines being up-ended; school and work turning virtual; dining out, parties, concerts, and vacations all vanishing into the vapor of memory. But for Matt and me, all of that sort of stuff turned out to be distracting fluff that coated, and often obscured, the ephemeral and precious thing that was Havi's existence with us. So many other things that usually seemed so important and consuming had turned out not to be at all.

For us, the past year was about making the most of time with Havi, and also, starting that June, with Kaia. It was about turning Havi's face to the sun and letting the wind chase itself through her golden curls. About daily walks and awaiting Havi's giggle to lift us through a day. About blueberries and challah. Family and some incredible friends. Welcoming another little girl into the world. Drinking in every little moment with Havi and forcing presence and present to be the only way to operate.

We will continue to love Havi in 2021, but it is anything but a happy new year for us. Soon we will lose her.

Although Havi has become very still and quiet, her presence in our lives is still immense—the kind of presence that only a child can claim as theirs. We know that when we lose her there will be a new quiet, a scary silence, and a hole in our hearts that will never be filled. For that hole is reserved for Havi, and only Havi. And the thing is, we can't know how that hole will change us. We just know it will. It already has.

So, this New Year's Day, as we celebrate Havi's fifty-fifth Shabbirthday, we sing to her, hold and rock her, and cherish another Friday with her in our arms.

Several days later, on Wednesday, January 6, 2021, we watch President-elect Joe Biden address the nation as a mob attacks the US Capitol. Of course, the magnitude of this moment doesn't register for Havi, and for that, I am grateful. But I also have to acknowledge to myself that I am struggling with cruelty and injustice right inside our home. I am feeling scared and lonely a lot too. And small and helpless.

CHAPTER 35

Holy Space

Matt and I soon settle back into our work routines; Tia and Kaia play all day; and Havi joins several Zoom calls with both Matt and me. I love having her with me—and I almost need her only an arm's length away.

But this morning, after I leave Havi with Tia during a particularly long call and make my way back upstairs to them, I find Tia crying. Havi is asleep in her arms in her bedroom rocking chair, having had a particularly challenging couple of days of eating. She chokes constantly, and labors through sucking and swallowing. Tia looks up at me as I enter the room. "How can these things happen to a child?" she asks, tears streaming down her cheeks. "Sometimes I'm angry. It's just, every day, she's losing more and more. It's impossible to watch. Also, it's even harder to be away from her."

I bend down and wrap my arms around both of them. "I know. It's impossible. I love you, T." And then I turn and walk out, closing the door gently behind me. I keep walking. I have to move. So I walk for forty-five minutes through our neighborhood.

Later that night, Matt and I call Charlie and Blyth. We stand by our dresser in our bedroom, with the phone on speaker. "Hi guys." Charlie and Blyth say in unison. Hearing their voice already empowers me.

"We've tried everything," I say. "I can't even get an ounce of smoothie into her. She just seals her lips and turns her head. I've tried a dozen times today, and she won't take anything." I speak with the biggest knot in my throat.

There is a long pause.

"She's ready," Blyth says softly and without hesitation. "She's been so clear and she's telling you. She's amazing. Just be with her. Let her lead you like you have for her whole life."

Charlie adds, "She's comfortable. I promise."

"How much time does she have left?" I ask.

"It could be a week, maybe less," Blyth says with a quiet conviction.

"Let's get her to the ocean," Matt says, turning toward me while we are still on the phone.

"That sounds exactly like where you should be," Charlie replies. And then, practically in unison, he and Blyth add, "We love you, call us with anything. We are here."

We hang up and turn toward each other. Matt pulls me in tight to his chest. We hold onto each other and cry.

"I'm not ready, Emmy," I say. "I thought I could be, but I'm not."

"I don't think we'll ever be ready. Let's go get her."

I walk into our bathroom and splash some water on my face, then follow Matt downstairs.

Matt calls Maggie and his parents, and tells them, "Come soon."

Havi is lying across her Aunt Leah and Aunt Erin on the living room couch. Uncle Jacob sits beside them rocking Kaia.

They look up at us, and from their eyes I know they want to ask us what Charlie and Blyth had said.

"Maybe a week," I tell them. "We should stop trying to feed her. She's ready."

They each look down at Havi and stroke her hair and rub her legs. I watch their eyes well with tears.

Matt and I sit down on the floor with our backs against the couch to feel Havi's skin against the back of our necks without disturbing her.

* * *

The next day, Matt and I walk over to my parents' apartment and tell them that Havi is getting ready to die. We sit across from them in their living room, with them on one couch, and us on the other.

"She doesn't want to drink any more smoothies. And we aren't going to intervene at all. We can't. She's ready," I say just above a whisper. It hurts to talk.

I look away. I can't make eye contact with my parents. I can practically hear their hearts breaking through the silence. My dad cries. My mom stands up to hold me. I let her.

"We're going to take her to the ocean tomorrow. Kaia will stay at home with Aunt Leah and Aunt Erin. We'll spend the night there and do some thinking about what we need these next few days," Matt says calmly.

"Whatever you need. We love you," my mom says.

"We're going to go home now to be with Havi," I say, turning toward the door.

After we close the door gently behind us, I look back through the window and see my parents holding each other, their bodies convulsing.

* * *

At home, we text the local posse and ask if we can talk to them that night. I send an unusually formal text message: "Let's meet in the front room at 8:00 p.m. so we can make a plan for the next few days."

They each arrive promptly. It is dark outside, and the living room space feels foreign and somber; we never gather here. We all stand together, and Matt and I tell them that Havi is dying, that she hasn't eaten now for the past two days, and that we need to listen to her. "She's ready to go soon," I say. "Aunt Maggie, Grandma, and Grandpa are on their way. And my parents know. We're going to the Cape tomorrow, to get Havi to the ocean one more time, and we're hoping you can all take care of Kaia while we're gone."

"We have one more ask," Matt says. "When we get back, we need each of you to treat this home as holy space. We know the doors are always open here, but this time is different now. We are in unchartered territory and we need space to listen to Havi closely, to hold her, to say goodbye. And we also want you to have time and space with her, but it needs to be on our terms. We're scared and don't know how to be right now, so just know how much we love you all."

"Also," Matt adds, "we're going to do some thinking about an intimate funeral service here, at home, after Havi dies. And we probably need your help."

I tell everyone we are going to head up to bed, and Matt and I turn and walk upstairs. Havi's posse is quiet. I'm not sure how long they stay in the front room, but I take comfort in knowing they have each other.

We get into bed, and Matt keeps his light on. "It's my turn this week, right?" "Yes, love. But we can do this one together if you want." "No, I want to write to her." And he opens his laptop and I fall asleep to the sound of his fingers striking the keyboard.

My Most Beautiful Girl,

Since the day we learned of your diagnosis we made a promise that we would listen closely to you.

Last weekend your mom and I sat and held you. You had changed a lot in a matter of just a few short days—or maybe it happened earlier and we just didn't see it. You've fooled us before—along with the rest of the medical establishment, for that matter. But now you've made it clear, several days in a row, that you aren't interested in the bottle and that eating has gotten harder, maybe too hard. And as your mom and I reckoned with this, you rested so peacefully held in Mom's arms, with your eyes closed and your beautiful head against her chest. You are just over two years old. How can it be that you have the mind to tell us when you are ready to die?

Sunday was a brilliant and cold day and I met Charlie in the morning for a walk at the Brookline public golf course. The course is closed for the season, save for the occasional hardy New England golfer, swinging solitarily in 25-degree weather, and that morning the course was quiet and filled with light. We followed the curving fairways and sloping greens as Charlie told me what the last days were like for Cameron, his daughter, and Hayden, his nephew, both of whom died of Tay-Sachs disease twenty years ago. He shared many things, including the beautiful story of a red-tailed hawk who visited Hayden during the week of his death and then later perched above his parents as they sat on Hayden's bench in New York's Central Park. As we came up on the ninth tee box, a red-tailed hawk glided close to the ground and across our path, landing on a low branch just ten yards away. The hawk turned its head and looked at us. It was close enough for me to see its pupils constrict and dilate as we came into its sharp focus.

On Monday, in the late afternoon, Mom and I took you back to that tree and I showed you both where that beautiful bird had sat and looked at us. As we stood there in the waning afternoon light, looking at that tree, it was as if Cameron and Hayden were saying to you, "Havi, you're with us now, beautiful girl." We talked with you a lot during that walk. And we listened to you and heard you. We won't push the bottle on you anymore. We'll stop making you go through those cracking, rasping, gurgling coughs when you try to eat, the sounds of which have echoed around the kitchen for so many days.

For someone who has never uttered a single word, your voice is so powerful and clear. We knew we had to get you back to the ocean. And so, on Wednesday morning, we left Kaia at home with Tia and Aunt Leah and Aunt E and threw some things in the car and drove down to Cape Cod, to Chatham and the coastline. We tucked you into your stroller and pushed you around the quiet town and down to the beach, which was windswept and empty and beautiful. It was a clear day, and warm by Boston's winter standards, and I felt serene and yet raw being near the water again with you. We kept you all wrapped up and maneuvered your stroller down the packed sand by the water's edge. Mostly you dozed, but you occasionally opened your beautiful eyes. "Hi, Havi girl!" your mom and I said. "Hi, beautiful girl!" We walked to the end and back again, leaving tracks of stroller wheels, footprints, and our tears.

Mom leaned in close to talk to you: "We don't get to plan so many things with you: birthdays, first days of the school year, your bat mitzvah, your wedding. But we will plan your funeral memorial with you, sweet Havi girl."

We awoke to a breathtaking sunrise back at home on your fifty-seventh Shabbirthday and took advantage of the warm sun to walk you up and down Heartbreak Hill in Newton. Mom narrated most of the way, talking you through some future Boston Marathon and making sure to point out where you two will start to pass people. After being outside with you nearly the whole day, Mom and I snuggled up with you on the downstairs couch and caught a short nap before dinner. Kaia spent most of the day with Tia at home again, but as soon as we walked back in the door with you, she couldn't wait to touch your cheeks and run her hands through your hair. Tia picked out a beautiful outfit for you, and you looked radiant. When we brought you downstairs, we found that your aunts and uncles had worked their magic again. The table was set with an array of lavender flowers, which capture so well the essence of you, and there were giant balloons spelling out "Havi 57" hung behind your chair. We ate all of your favorite meals—most importantly, blueberry pancakes—and made sure to hold some of the sweet blueberries against your lips so you could taste them. And we kissed you and hugged you and passed you around from one set of arms to another.

You have a number of days remaining now. The pain of losing you feels different, scarier and stronger. We used to fear all the things we'd have to stop doing together, but now we are overcome by the fear of just not being with you. We've always dreaded this moment—the moment when you would tell us you were ready. But now we are afraid for having to live the rest of our lives without you. We wish we could go with you wherever you're going. Of course, we know you'll somehow still be with us wherever we are. But please don't be shy about just coming right in, coming back home whenever you can, whenever you want.

If this is the last time we write to you in this way, we want you to know that we will spend the rest of our lives figuring out all the ways we can carry you on with us, and remember and honor you. Fridays will forever be yours.

Saturday mornings, too. We are so scared to feel far away from you.

We love you. We already miss you and we always will.

Love,

Dad

CHAPTER 36

January 20, 2021

In the days leading up to January 20, the weather feels more like early spring—Havi days, full of soft light and luminous sky from sunrise to sunset. We bundle her up and take her for long walks every day, drinking "Havi chocolates" along the way, retracing our usual loop through the trees and meadows of the silent golf course.

I sit with Havi on my lap, her mouth open and her lips wrapped around my nose. I can see the gentle rise and fall of her chest and hear her breathing. Her breath is the only thing keeping her in this life, as opposed to the place she will be in the coming days. We are in her white rocking chair in her bedroom. This is where she taught me how to become a mother. She was patient with me as I learned to breastfeed; she tested my patience when she'd resist sleep; she'd make me relax when her fingers strummed my arm or my belly; and she stretched my heart in every direction when she smiled and cooed.

> Hav, when we would read together and I'd watch you turn the pages of *Goodnight Moon*, I felt like it was only a matter of time before you'd be teaching me things you'd learn in school. I imagined you and Dad talking circles around me about science and medicine one day. We daydreamed together in this chair about the way things should have been. We cried together in this chair a lot too, for totally different reasons, but our tears are all over it. Your spit-up is too. That's only right because this is our sacred place. It's where I have looked so deeply into your biggest eyes and couldn't believe that Dad and I had actually made someone so beautiful. Where I pressed my cheek against yours and could never find the words to describe how soft and delicious that felt.

Where I sat and watched you and Dad dance together before bed or kept him company throughout the night as he rocked you back to sleep in a way that only he could do.

This is our place, where we looked out the window together and saw the seasons change. Where we waited for Tia to come scoop you up so I could rush off to work. Where I'd sit with you and your aunts and uncles and laugh and cry. Where all of your friends and family got to spend magical time with you, and where you shared your love and wisdom with them.

This sacred white rocking chair is where we first discovered your startle reflex, where you learned to hold your bottle by yourself, where we held you through seizures, and where, last night, we gave you your last dose of Keppra mixed with a few drops of smoothie. And now, it's where we listen to Dad's sobs downstairs as he pours the remainder of your final bottle down the kitchen sink. And this is also where we'd say goodnight to you and then gently place you in your rocker so you could sleep comfortably. Where I'd hold you and Kaia together and imagine the two of you running in and out of each other's rooms. This chair, our place, has held everything—the biggest love and the deepest pain. And so, let's plan to meet back in your chair whenever you're up for it, whenever you want to return.

The feelings inside your dad and me are different now. The fear of losing you, the difficulty of watching you lose everything, the anger at the life that Tay-Sachs was stealing, and now has stolen from us—all of that has been replaced by a consuming ache, a pounding pain that is the realization that soon you will be physically gone from our lives forever. Forever. And now all we want is to have you back. Just for a minute, even only for a second. We feel physically battered and bruised and the emptiness is so heavy. I want to hold your warm body and rub our faces against your impossibly soft cheeks. I want to watch Dad squeeze you just a little too hard and hear your full-bodied sigh once he lets go. I want to watch him brush his lips back and forth across yours and see you turn your head back and forth, mirroring his.

The way we carry you from now until forever matters. We will always want to talk about you, and we will only talk about you in the most tender, loving way. We will ask others to do the same. You are not a secret. You are not merely a beautiful memory. You are our beautiful, oldest daughter who we will honor and cherish forever and who will live on through our love for you and for each other.

We have shared you. We had no choice, really. But it's a good thing. From the moment you arrived, your incredible family and friends scooped you up and never let you go. They took you everywhere. They made you feel like an absolute queen. They gave you everything— thoughtful gifts, delicious treats. But mostly they gave you a big, crazy love that is totally unparalleled. With them, you never seemed sick. With them, we got more of you. We got to see you through their eyes. And they are all aching now with us, Beauty.

So today, and forever, we will honor you with them. Your people. I love you.

* * *

The house has been transformed into holy space now. Havi is on day six of no sustenance and her breathing has started to change. For the last twenty-four hours, Havi, Matt, and I have been moving between her room and our bed listening to the songs that have played on repeat over the last year. Our closest posse has assembled quietly and I can hear them talking in low voices in the kitchen and living room. This evening, we bring Havi down to the kitchen for one last dance party and pass her around to all of her aunts and uncles, each of them selecting their own special song to share their last dance. Matt and I get the final song with her, and choose Cole Swindell's "You Should Be Here," and the three of us sway together and press our faces against hers.

We walk upstairs with Havi in our arms, and into our bedroom so she can be next to us because we aren't sure she will even make it through the night. She starts to moan. Her breathing becomes irregular. Matt gets the morphine and drips a little of the bright blue liquid into her cheek. He picks her up. Her body is limp. He rests her head gently on his pillow. And for the rest of the night, Matt and I rotate sides so that we can stare at her face. Every couple of hours, her moaning starts, and Matt gives her a few more drops of the morphine.

Now, morning is here. Wednesday, January 20, 2021.

The three of us lay folded together in our bed like an origami swan: Havi's tiny body motionless on mine, her head limp on my chest, her legs straddling my hips. Matt's forehead is pressed against mine. His arms are wrapped around Havi and me. The room is still, silent except for the beating of each of our hearts.

I feel like the three of us are having an unspoken conversation. I stare so deeply into Havi's eyes, trying to intuit what she wants us to know before she leaves the physical world forever. Then I hear her. I turn to Matt and say, "I think she's telling you not to hide. That you are too smart and creative and loving to hide in this house for the rest of your life. And that she wants you and us to really live in the world."

"Don't hide," Matt repeats out loud, as he holds Havi's tiny, fragile hands in his. Then he turns to me: "Of course she'd say that. Because all I want to do is hide."

At 9:04 a.m., Havi takes her last breath against my chest with Matt wrapping both of us in his arms. She is two years, four months, and sixteen days old.

A small movement at the window draws my and Matt's eyes. A tiny, gray stinkbug crawls over the molding. It pauses, staring at Matt, Havi and me from across the room.

Havi sent us a stinkbug. "Seriously, Havi girl?" I say, barely above a whisper. Matt and I break into laughter that quickly dissolves into tears.

Embrace the mystery. Hold each other. Laugh. Snuggle a lot. Vow to live life to its fullest. And when it's time, get out of bed and save the stinkbug.

* * *

Matt and I make the decision to keep Havi's body in our home, in her room for a few days before taking her to the funeral home. We bathe her and dress her in a dark blue and lavender onesie. We place her stiff and cold body in her rocker, with her head resting between two stuffies, rossie the rhino, and mr. otter. Throughout each day, I visit her there. Her spirit is close by but has certainly left her body; it happened so fast. When I close her bedroom door, I feel like we can talk privately, though. I hate it. And I need this time. Somehow I wonder if with every conversation, with each tear, I am gently guiding her to wherever she's already headed.

We hold a small, private funeral service held in our living room, that includes a few words from each member of Havi's family-friend posse. We don't yet know how we'll honor her with our full community, but we want to do something while she is still physically with us. Leah and Erin organize an intimate and sacred service, and each of us share a few words about Havi. We also ask everyone to write a letter to Kaia. We want her to have them to read some day.

The next day, Grandi and Grandadders pick Kaia up for a morning walk so that Matt and I can say our last goodbye to Havi's body in her room and prepare to take her to the funeral home. I pick her up and bring her downstairs. I walk slowly with Havi's body in my arms, until I can't anymore. My legs give out and I feel Matt's arms around me helping to hold me up. I sob, and close my eyes, and scrunch my nose. I am not sure I'll be able to let go of her. But then I do. I place her gently in the beautiful wicker basket lined with lavender cloth. We form a half-circle; Matt and me with our posse, all standing around Havi's body resting peacefully in folds of lavender at the bottom of the stairs. I lock eyes with my brother. For the first time I see fear in them. *Where do we go from here?* I am scared as hell.

We carry her out to our car and place the basket on the folded-down seats of our Jeep. Our posse caravans behind us.

We arrive at the funeral home. I don't know how to say goodbye. But eventually, I walk out of there and we drive to the beach.

PART
IV

"... 'Tis a human thing, love,
A holy thing, to love
What death has touched."

YEHUDA HALEVI

CHAPTER 37

Holy Wednesdays

Once Havi is gone, Wednesday becomes her day. She died on a Wednesday, so that day now has a permanent Havi mark. Matt and I meditate in her room. We spend time walking outside. We cry. We study photographs. We reread letters from our people. We listen to the music that reminds us of her and helps to evoke her memory. If she were still here, if she were healthy, we know that we would devote far more than one day per week to care and love and pay attention to our first daughter, so setting aside one day per week to turn our attention toward her in a meaningful and sacred way feels like the only way to make it through a week. We keep writing, too.

On that first Wednesday, January 27, 2021, without Havi, Matt writes to her.

> Hi Beauty,
>
> I can't believe it's been a week. I can't believe you're gone. Forever. There are moments where the rhythm of a day lulls me into thinking that I'm going to come up to your room and see you resting peacefully in your rocker by the window; moments when the quiet of the house feels like it did when you were with us; there are moments when I tell myself you're on a walk with Tia because it's the only way to get through a part of the day. But you are gone now. How can that be?
>
> Most days are filled with a bizarre and meaningless array of activities. I feel like I am walking in circles, moving things around on one shelf in the kitchen, wandering off to some other room, and then moving all of those things back again. My friend Jesse and I organized batteries, audited the miscellaneous cable bin, hung pictures, and then did it all

again. Mom spends most of her days in your room, sitting in your chair, writing in her journal, and nursing and loving Kaia. And then, all of a sudden, it's dinnertime, and then we're off to sit in bed and talk and remember.

We've all been spending a lot of time in your room. It still smells like you and the warmth from the sun coming in through the window feels like you. Your rocker is still exactly as you left it, with the pajamas you died in resting in between your two stuffed animals, Rossi the Rhino that Uncle Jacob and Aunt Erin brought you from their honeymoon, and the seal from Chatham that you snuggled with during your final trip to the beach.

So, what happens now? We take some additional time off, get your room in order, eat our way through the fifth tray of Jewish desserts that kind friends have sent to us and then just go back to our normal, humdrum lives? That feels so wrong.

We're headed to the beach soon for our second Shabbirthday without you. It's Uncle Jacob's thirty-fifth birthday this weekend. We've packed our clothes, Kaia's clothes, Kaia's travel crib, the space heater, and the sound machine. But it feels like we're traveling too light. All we want to do is add your rocker, medicines, bottles, blankets into the mix if it means we can undo last Wednesday.

You should be here.

Where are you? Do you think you could come back soon?

Dad

* * *

By early February, yet another week further away from the last time we held Havi, the weather changes dramatically. It is grayer and colder outside. Sometimes it feels like maybe Havi knew it was about to get gross out and decided to head south or west for the winter. If that is the case, I want her to get some extra sun for me.

I spend most hours of most days sitting in Havi's rocking chair. Her aunts string two long rows of photos, clipped onto a piece of brown twine, on the wall and I sit looking at them. They show her smiling, sleeping, laughing, cuddling—and each one is more compelling than the next. It is easy to lose myself in these photos, as I try desperately to remember the sounds, smells, and feelings from each photographed moment. Havi's room is safe and peaceful. I fill jars with her Aveeno soap, Dreft detergent, fancy hotel shampoos and calendula lotion so that her room smells like her. With the shade open, it is warm and bright and alive in a way that feels so much like Havi's spirit. I am not sure what I believe yet about where she is, but I could feel her in here.

Oh, but of course it isn't the same as having her with me. It doesn't even come close. I had no idea how much I'd ache for her body against mine, how every cell in my body is programmed to hold her, feed her, walk with her, bathe her, cuddle and sleep with her. Without her, my body feels empty, confused, neglected, disoriented. My movements feel unnatural. I forget which way to turn when I walk out of my room; my arms ache without her in them; I wonder how I'll sing her to sleep without her warm body against my chest; I cross and uncross my legs at the kitchen table, trying to remember how to sit without her between my knees. I outline her hair and her face in the air with my fingers. When I close my eyes tightly, I can almost feel her. But *almost* has never felt so big. The presence of her absence[1] fills the spaces where she used to be; the presence of her absence, that is what we live with now.

"It's so big, isn't it? The presence of her absence," Dr. Jo says to us the first time we speak to her after Havi dies. "As soon as I heard your voices, I could feel it all the way across the country." She is right. Havi's absence is everywhere. And I hate it. I hate what her absence represents. The permanence. How quiet and dull her absence feels, compared to the real her. I hate that we are robbed of any future with her and that we somehow have to adjust to her absence. I don't want to adjust to it. I only want her back.

That first week after Havi dies, I run one afternoon through the arboretum, the nearby 281-acre public park with thousands of plants and dozens of trails to explore. I stay on the trails that are mostly hidden from

---

[1] See Joanne Cacciatore, *Bearing the Unbearable: Love, Loss and the Heartbreaking Path of Grief* (Somerville, MA: Wisdom Publications, 2017).

the walking paths. I don't want to see other people, especially people who don't know Havi. Strangers. They feel unsympathetic and cold and represent to me the world moving on without Havi in it. It starts to snow. Instinctively, I stick my tongue out to try and catch a flake, and I smile. Havi loved to do that. She pulls me out of my bitterness and self-pity and brings a smile to my face.

Later that day, when I return from my run, I shower, and then sit in Havi's room to write. I am on my third journal now. Writing allows me to connect, visit, integrate Havi into my days. It keeps her in the front row of my life. Where she belongs. And I want to write for Kaia too. So that maybe one day she will read all about this crazy, tragic, and beautiful time of our lives. Only if she wants.

I am reading a lot, too, trying to make sense of what I feel and believe. I read only what Dr. Jo recommends on her website's reading list, and anything that Charlie and Blyth suggest. Francis Weller's *Wild Edge of Sorrow*, John O'Donohue's *Bless the Space Between Us*, and Mitch Albom's *Tuesdays with Morrie*. I read one and then turn to another of the three, over and over. That combination of grief literature, poetry, and memoir helps me understand my grief and gives me language for my feelings. Language enables me to educate others on real-life grief. This is empowering.

I make a blueberry smoothie every morning. I like hearing the familiar sound of the blender, and I like how it makes me feel like I am still taking care of Havi, nourishing her somehow. We minimize the importance of continuing bonds in American culture, I think in part because it makes us feel too deeply, and in doing so, it throws into question our very being. But without such rituals, we risk losing connection to those we can't see anymore. And I am not going to do that—not with my daughter. So I make her a blueberry smoothie just as I had when she was still with us, only a few weeks earlier, and I trust that I am not crazy for doing it.

Kaia doesn't sleep well that first week after Havi dies, and Matt and I are exhausted from staying up with her. She is missing Havi too, yearning for her big sister without the language to express it. She plays in Havi's room, crawls onto her rocking chair, and stares at Havi's photos for long stretches of time. My heart breaks watching Kaia grieving with us, and I trust that missing Havi is far healthier than minimizing Havi's passing. Or pretending her away.

So we decide that, at least for the time being, we will keep Havi alive in the only ways we can, through placing photographs of her throughout the house, enjoying blueberry smoothies and muffins every morning, displaying bouquets of purple flowers, listening to Havi's favorite music, and keeping up our weekly Shabbirthday ritual. These powerful reminders become a lesson to us that we rely on every day: Symbols, colors, and meaningful physical manifestations of the people we've lost help us send our love for them out into the world. They serve as a reminder that they existed, they still exist, their energy cannot be destroyed.

CHAPTER 38

Both/And

Matt and I return to work on February 9, twenty days after losing Havi. Twenty days feels like no time at all, and yet, I am grateful. In the US, there are currently no nationwide laws that require employers to provide employees either paid or unpaid leave after a death. This is criminal. We do not go back to work because we want a "distraction" or a "break" from our grief, though. We'd never want that. Grief is now a part of who we are, and a way for Matt and me to be with Havi. And grief doesn't have to be scary or sad at all—it is powerful and lifesaving.

If the world saw grieving people as beautiful, sacred, and strong, instead of scary, weak, and sad, offering and receiving compassion would feel very different. Grieving, I am learning, is a way to continue to express our love and devotion to Havi, a way to keep her close in a most surreal yet completely natural part of parenting. Her death is anachronistic and traumatic, and devastating. I hate that she isn't here physically. I want to actually go find her as I write this. And yet, grieving is my way forward. It is the way I transform my longing into some semblance of a new life. It is my way of being that is real and raw and enduring.

We return to work because we have to. We need to stay connected to other parts of our lives, to earn a living, and to have some structure to our days. We request flexibility on Wednesdays—Havi days—and our employers grant us that, so we know we can count on those days to reconnect with Havi and take care of each other and ourselves. Most importantly, we don't subscribe to the "time will heal" mantra, so we are not about following a grief timeline, despite the pressure from the external world to do so. We get messages from people who mean well, saying things like, "It must feel good to be distracted at work." Or, "You're through the worst of it." Or "Kaia must be so helpful to have in the house." But no. No. No. These messages are not helpful—in some cases, they are in fact harmful. No, I don't want to be distracted from Havi—I want to remember her. And no, we are not through the worst of it. Havi is not here anymore, and we are only at the beginning of her absence from our lives.

And, of course, Kaia is and will always be a gift. Our love for her is beyond measure. And she is Kaia. She isn't Havi. And it isn't her responsibility to make us feel better. Perhaps more helpful comments would have been: "I can imagine returning to work feels disorienting. I'm here if you want to talk. I love you." Or: "I saw the most beautiful purple flower today and thought of Havi. I am with you as you make this transition back to work." Or: "I can imagine caring for Kaia is incredible, exhausting, and confusing. I wish she still had her big sister here, too. Love you."

Our first Havi day, after returning to work, falls in February. Matt and I spend a slow morning in Havi's room, listening to her playlist, meditating, and looking through photos to print. Then we go for a long and therapeutic run in the arboretum. I lead Matt through snow-covered trails that he has never been on. It is quiet and so bright, with the sun reflecting off the snow. I notice Matt's tongue sticking out. After a quick lunch back home, we grab our coats and leave once again, this time to drive out to Manchester-by-the-Sea, to Singing Beach, which is where we sought refuge after bringing Havi to the funeral home. We turn on Havi's playlist, and drive in silence for forty-five minutes. We arrive. The brilliant sunshine pours out of the crisp blue sky. The clouds are wispy streaks and there is a pull in the air that brings us toward the water. The sand is covered in white snow down to the tideline, where waves have left a smooth edge marking the transition from our terrestrial world to the other place in the sea. Matt and I stand at that threshold for a long time, looking out over the Atlantic, straining to see into the other dimension.

"Snow on sand," Matt reaches for my hand. "In my mind those two elements don't exist together. Wow. Kind of crazy beautiful."

Seagulls fly overhead, and the wind chases itself in circles, looking for Havi's curls. I squeeze Matt's hand. "Am I crazy for thinking I'd see her out here?"

"No. Of course not. You are her mom."

We write her name in the sand with our feet. We love seeing her name. Then we watch the waves wash her name away again, and we walk hand-in-hand back to the car.

On the way home from the beach, we talk about learning to exist in a "both/and" way that lets us experience all the most painful feelings of missing Havi and at the same time live a joyful, rich, expansive life. The rest of the world, or at least the rest of our Western world, doesn't seem to know how to do that very well.

* * *

Hi Peanut,

It's Dad again.

How can it be that you left this physical world four weeks ago? The time has gone by too fast. Or rather, I hate that the number of days from when I last held you in my arms continues to increase. There are still moments, faint and hazy, in every day when I wander close to the expectation that I'll hold you again; that you're in your room or out on a walk and that you'll be back soon. And then my hyper-rational mind snaps me back to the reality that you are gone. It's confusing. It's consuming.

I've had the inclination this week to call my best friends but I've stopped short before dialing their numbers. When I imagine them picking up the phone, I realize that I don't have much to say. I don't have the language to explain the feelings, the struggle, the pain. And then I'm left feeling like I read out loud a few lines of a greeting card to describe the most intense and agonizing experience of my life. So it's better to walk with those feelings alone where they can marinate and burn in their indescribable tastes and colors. Maybe at some point I'll be able to wade back into the pool of "normal" society, but from where I am standing now it looks mighty muted and dull, full of trivial daily anxieties, consumption with superficial and meaningless milestones of work and wealth. Whereas the world with Havi, and without her, exists on a wholly different plane, where time is a physical dimension and meaning in a day is defined by the feeling of sun on your face and the sound of the wind in your ears.

Dad

* * *

The following morning, I sit in Havi's chair with Kaia in my lap, and notice that outside the window the sun pokes through the clouds. Its light and warmth draw my gaze toward the outdoors, to the branches outside covered in a sparkling fresh snow and the clouds that move through the sky like Havi: slowly, beautifully, with a numinous splendor. Havi draws Matt outside early in the mornings, too. It has been snowing a lot lately, and Matt has taken to shoveling as soon as he's awake. He visits with Havi out there, he tells me. This morning, sitting in Havi's room with Kaia, I hear the sound of Matt's snow shovel scraping in rhythm on the driveway. I carry Kaia to the window to peek out at him. As he moves his body, I imagine Havi perched on his shoulders, pointing to the next spot he should clean up. Kaia and I tap on the window, and Matt looks up at us.

"Do you see Dad out there?" I whisper in Kaia's ear.

"Hi Kaia, I see you!" Matt responds with a full-face smile and waves up at us.

Kaia waves back so fiercely, and smiles with her whole body. She can wave now. This is a big deal. I see Matt's shoulders relax and how his smile matches hers. Then, even from all the way upstairs and through a window, I see tears in his eyes. And I feel my own well up, too. Without a word, we know: *Havi should be here too.* In her snowsuit, outside with Matt, laughing in the cold, teaching her little sister how to shovel. Every single day we will have to grieve these losses. There is no timeline for grief.

CHAPTER 39

Soul Spark

Toward the end of February, the daily delivery of notes and flowers and food slows down. It has been a month, after all, since we lost Havi, and the world beyond our inner circle has started to move beyond her. Our bubble remains strong, though. The Sibs and Grandi and Grandadders still live only a mile away, and every night we have at least six people for dinner at our kitchen table. Kaia lives in a full house.

On a Wednesday morning in the middle of February, I sit in Havi's room on a Zoom call with my parent's rabbi in Philadelphia. I feel pulled toward spirituality and safe with Rabbi Shelly, as she knows and loves my family. During our call, she shares a concept from a book by Melinda Ribner called *New Age Judaism: Ancient Wisdom for the Modern World*. It applies to the way our family has supported us in keeping Havi's memory alive, and it's this: "that a great soul usually reincarnates not in a single body but in many people. This increases the likelihood of that soul accomplishing its mission in this lifetime. In such cases, a number of people contain sparks from the very same soul."[1] You all have Havi's soul spark in you, Rabbi Shelly explains. I listen. Maybe we do. And maybe we need her spark to continue to grow into better versions of ourselves—the versions she'd be most proud of, especially as our longing for her intensifies. Sharing memories about the people we've lost reinforces that their life mattered, and still matters, and makes their loss less ambiguous. They can exist both psychologically and in our physical world this way.

* * *

From the earliest time I can remember, I attended Hebrew school on Thursdays and Sundays. *Tikkun Olam*, the Hebrew phrase meaning

---

[1] Melinda Ribner, *New Age Judaism: Ancient Wisdom for the Modern World* (Deerfield Beach, FL: Simcha Press/Health Communications, 2000), 156.

"repair of the world," was an ever-present thread woven throughout our Reconstructionist-Conservative Jewish education, and always resonated with me. My family attended Beth Am Israel Synagogue, where, as Reconstructionists, we approached Judaism and life with deep devotion to the past and a passion for and insistence on relating it to the present. Our teachers invited us to find relevance and present-day meanings in *Divrei Torah* (Torah commentaries), which helped us draw lessons from Torah texts. For example, when we read the book of Exodus story of the Israelites being about to cross the Red Sea, we'd discuss questions like: What did you have to believe to cross the Red Sea? Who might be apprehensive about crossing? How does a leader help in a moment like this?

Our rabbi and cantor both encouraged us to embrace the mystical elements of our lives, those things which allowed us to feel connected to the divine. As a kid, I took this to mean that there is something bigger than ourselves. I thought maybe G-d was the goodness in each of us—the part that we can access when we are feeling loved and safe, and when we serve others. Compassion, courage, and forgiveness were among the values we pulled out of weekly Torah readings. Jewish education was also about taking action, being responsible—it was not about blindly following anything or anyone.

I was a kid, though, and only rarely could I appreciate the depth and import of what was going on within the four walls of my Hebrew school class. So, what really kept me engaged were the soft pretzels for snack time and the epic games of tag that we sneaked in during breaks.

I do not want to under- or overstate the role that Hebrew school played in my life. It was simply a part of my weekly routine that continued even while I was devoted to soccer and basketball. I wasn't sure back then exactly what Judaism meant to me, but I knew that the teachings aligned with what I felt in my heart about community: It is not only a place, it is also an evolving, growing web of connection, learning, and shared experience that allows us to live life with a fuller sense of love, empathy, and purpose. And I saw a direct connection between Hebrew school and team sports, too. In sports and at Hebrew school I saw how something incredibly powerful, even beyond articulation, happens when people care about others before themselves, when there is an appreciation of differences, and when we have to dig deep into our souls to find another gear.

*   *   *

Matt spins. We don't post our entries on CaringBridge, but we continue to write. He isn't sharing much with me these days, so opening our journal and reading his entry is my best window into his head and heart. I worry about him.

February 26, 2021

Hi Sweet Girl,

I don't like life without you here. We are trying to make the best of it. Writers tell us to explore our grief, for there is beauty in it. They say that love and loss are infinitely woven together and that the fullest heart is a broken one. Maybe that's true. But none of these words that I write will bring you back, which is all I really want.

What happened to the life we were supposed to have with you? What happened to the sound of your giggle floating across space, the one that seemed to play on repeat throughout the day? What happened to me always having to catch my breath a little when your sparkling eyes locked with mine? And how can it be that your impossibly soft skin and golden curls feel so far away, Peanut? For the last two years, and especially for the past year, you were with us for every waking minute of every day. And for most of those minutes you were in our arms. We fed you every bite of food, held the straw to your lips for every sip, rocked you to sleep every night, and breathed our breaths alongside yours. Our days and your days were like a beautiful secret dance, choreographed perfectly so.

And then in one fleeting moment all of that was gone. So quickly your rhythm disappeared from our life. I feel like I'm flailing, and failing, to get it back. Somehow I put one foot in front of the other and get through each day, but in those movements I am numb.

I am sitting in your room as I write, on another Saturday morning. We're in an interim time, where no place looks like itself, as the late poet John O'Donohue puts it.

We love you, beauty. Be patient with us during this in-between time.

Dad

CHAPTER 40

Finding Motion

March 30, 2021. Havi is gone for two months and ten days. Kaia is nine months old.

The sharp rap on our front door is the sound I've been waiting for. I hand Kaia to Tia, throw the door open, and lug the package off the porch and into the house. "It's your Baby Einstein walker," I tell nine-month-old Kaia.

As I cut open the box and unpack the walker, Kaia can barely contain herself. Hands outstretched, legs kicking, she tries to jump out of Tia's arms. Tia sets Kaia down on the kitchen floor. Kaia grips the walker's handlebar, pulls herself upright, pushes the walker two steps in my direction, and beams up at me. I crouch, facing her, grinning back at my second daughter. Then I start to cry. Sisters are not supposed to be severed from one another. With Kaia's every wobbly step, I imagine Havi's gentle hands guiding her, a sight I'll never see. Still, I feel Havi close, cheering Kaia on in her own way, from her own place in the universe.

* * *

Now that we're both working full time again, Matt and I need our Wednesday date-days more than ever. On this unusually warm March day—sunny, fifty degrees—we head for Newton, the neighboring suburb. After a brief stop for energy chews for our ten-mile run, training for the second annual Havi Half Marathon in May, we start with a slow trot down Commonwealth Avenue. *Thank you, Hav,* I think as I jog, *for teaching Dad and me to take the time for a long run in the middle of the workweek on a beautiful day in March. Thank you for keeping us anchored to what matters most; for teaching us to be present. Prioritize the people you love. Chase the sun.*

As we're running, Matt tells me the dream he had the night before. "I got to hold Havi, My. She smiled so big at me, and I scooped her up. Then she laid in my arms."

"I'm jealous," I admit.

"Don't be. I was so angry when I woke up and she was gone."

"At least you got to be with her."

"Not the point, My."

We run the next few miles in silence.

I listen to the rhythmic tap of our shoes on pavement, to Matt's shallowing breathing. For us running is a meditative practice. It opens our minds, our hearts, and our souls; makes us closer to what's real and raw in us. Even when it doesn't feel good, I know it strengthens our capacity to cope. As Dr. Jo says, "it gets harder before you get stronger."

"Want to keep talking, Emmy?" I ask Matt.

"No, Love," he answers.

The two of us have lost a bit of our rhythm. It doesn't feel good.

I remind myself that Matt and I are going through a transformation, or transfiguration, as O'Donohue calls it. I remind myself that this is never linear, never easy. We have to trust—in this moment, I have to trust—that if we stay with the pain and the confusion, we'll emerge stronger, better able to carry Havi with us for the rest of our lives, better able to raise Kaia so that she, too, gets to experience this fullness of love and spirit. I don't know how to do any of this. So all I can do is keep writing, and keep running.

*   *   *

Matt and I run another ten miles this week in preparation for the Havi Half. We run in our neighborhood along roads we've walked hundreds of times with Havi. We include a "quiet mile," from mile seven to eight. We don't speak to each other. We run gently, contemplatively, intentionally turning toward Havi. After we are a quarter mile into mile eight, Matt breaks our silence. "Where'd you go just now?"

"No place good," I say.

*   *   *

Havi's physical absence is everywhere. It lives inside me, sometimes as a dull ache in my back or tension in my neck. In the shower I feel her failing, slippery body against mine. I smell her in my blueberry smoothie every morning; I reach to support her at the dinner table every night; I strain to hear her when I close my book at night and try and sleep; I extend my hand across the empty seat as I sit between it and Kaia in the back seat of the car. Havi follows me throughout my workday, greeting me between Zoom meetings when I run upstairs to give Kaia a hug and peer into the empty rocker in her own room.

Whenever I sit in her absence, in quiet and solitude, her spirit visits me. Havi's spirit looks like a collage of her smiles and big eyes. It sounds like a video montage of her silliest giggles and sweetest coos. It wraps me in her soft skin and delicate arms. Sometimes Havi's spirit moves me to smile or cry or laugh out loud. Other times, it makes me talk out loud to her—to tell her that I'm doing okay and invite her to visit if she wants to.

I tend to look upward whenever I speak to Havi, although I don't really imagine her in the sky. I imagine her back in my belly, getting a second chance at this life.

The intensity of these moments takes my breath away and leaves me exhausted. But they are also the moments that make living feel worthwhile. When I question the value of going on, it's not so much that I want to die. It's that I want to be with Havi. When I say this to Dr. Jo, she says, "Yes, of course." She is not afraid of my feelings. And neither am I.

CHAPTER 41

Cornville

Sometime in the spring, we begin a ritual with Kaia of saying good morning to Havi in the many photographs we have of her in our bedroom. The ritual ends with Kaia planting a big, wet *beso* on Havi's lips in the photograph on our dresser. That seems to be the one she likes best. She stretches out her arms and reaches for Havi, brings the photograph close to her, locks eyes with Havi's, and then pushes her lips down against the glass. Meanwhile, I place my right hand on my heart, to hold their love for each other, and my left one on my stomach to try and steady myself because it never ceases to shock me that Kaia cannot kiss the living version of her sister. Then Matt and I take Kaia downstairs for breakfast.

At breakfast, Kaia barely sits in her highchair long enough to eat three Cheerios. Then she's off to circle time in a corner of our kitchen with her stuffed animal friends—Slippery Seal, Mr. Moose, Mr. Dog, Ms. Unicorn, and Mr. Avocado. Each had belonged to Havi, and now they are Kaia's, and she loves being with them as Matt makes up a circle time routine for her every morning.

We miss talking with Dr. Jo for the first half of April because she is away for four weeks, tending to her dying brother. Now Matt and I talk to her from Volante Farms after finishing a replenishing run, seated in the same spot where we had a picnic with Havi for her second birthday. It feels good to hear her voice and talk with her about the depths of grief without having to explain or defend or justify how we feel. She lets us be in the darkest part of our missing and aching, without minimizing or colonizing our feelings.

Matt starts to describe to Dr. Jo the overwhelming sense we've been having that there is something beyond us on earth that we can't explain. He stops mid-sentence, and then interrupts himself. "Holy shit. A red-tailed hawk is just hanging in the air above us." In a prior life, I would have dismissed the moment as sheer serendipity. Or, more likely, I wouldn't have even noticed. But now, I embrace the mystery. While I know that Havi isn't that red-tailed hawk, I allow myself to believe that the hawk arrives to reassure us that our souls and Havi's soul have found each other again. Even just for a moment.

During our phone call, we solidify plans to visit Dr. Jo at her Carefarm in Cornville, Arizona, where she has a respite house for traumatically bereaved families. Shortly after Havi dies, Dr. Jo suggests that we visit, as she thinks it will be a good idea for us to spend a few days with her in person, going deeper with our grief exploration and experiencing a therapeutic place where we'd feel safe and close to Havi. It takes us a few months to find a window of time where we feel comfortable leaving Kaia in the care of Tia, the Sibs, and Grandi and Grandadders, but now everything is set.

* * *

So on a Thursday morning, we leave our home for the first time in a year, to visit Dr. Jo's Carefarm. Matt is anxious about leaving Kaia behind. He is nervous about leaving the comfort and safety of our routines. He dreads being away from our house, where Havi is still so present. In fact, had it been up to him we may not have gone, but I feel so strongly about it he defers to me.

"Don't hide." I channel Havi as we prepare for our trip. It is from her that I have the strength and conviction to get on an airplane and travel across the country.

Tia arrives early in the morning to be with Kaia, and soon afterward, Jacob drives Matt and me to the airport. When we arrive in Phoenix, we rent a car and make the nearly two-hour drive up Interstate 17 to Cornville. It doesn't take long for us to get out of metropolitan Phoenix, where desert gives way to rolling hills and mesas and finally we crest into the red-striped mountains encircling Cornville.

The Carefarm faces west, looking toward the Woodchute Mountain range, which appears at times throughout the day like a dark silhouette against the bright blue sky. The Selah guest house, our respite place, is to our right as we drive in, next to a small reflection pond and a cozy, wooden, one-room cabin that houses an art studio. The main house, down the hill, is set in the middle of a series of green pastures where Dr. Jo's rescued horses, donkeys, goats, and alpacas roam.

Dr. Jo walks up the dirt road barefoot next to the high white fence of the horse pasture in jeans and a black tank top. Her long, dark hair is pulled back into a braid that shows off the tattoos on her back and arms. When she gets close enough, she greets us with huge hugs and the same slow "Hiiiii Myra, Hiiiii Matt" that we heard on the phone so many times before. This is the first time we lay eyes on each other. And yet, it feels like we've met a million times before. She tours us around the farm. We meet the dogs—Percy, Aspen, Lu, and Athena—and the goats, who are so funny and loving. They all trail Dr. Jo like babies following their mother, with Marta, Dr. Jo's favorite goat, leading the way. Dr. Jo shows us the back pasture, the circle swing, and the yoga deck by the river. It is an amazing place—Dr. Jo's husband Dave calls it "an amusement park of grief."

The natural world is on full display here, and Matt and I find some incredible running trails and dirt roads. We run very early each morning and watch the sun come up over the mountains. When we get back, I pump. I want to make sure I sustain my breastmilk supply for Kaia. I wonder how Havi and Kaia would like it here.

Dr. Jo wanders over to the respite house in the mid-morning, and we spend three or four hours talking. "Start wherever you'd like," she says. In one session, Dr. Jo describes our current state as a process of "deconstructing and reconstructing" our lives. Havi has changed us forever, and the reconstruction will be more full, more beautiful, more alive than how we lived before. But it will also forever be missing an essential piece. We break for lunch, and then get back together in the afternoon for some mindfulness practices in the form of painting rocks, barefoot walking, yoga, and meditation. Our days are filled fully inhabiting our grief.

On our final morning together, Dr. Jo leads us in meditation. We start by listening quietly to the world around us and to all of the layers of each sound. "Get underneath each sound," she tells us. Then Dr. Jo invites us to go to a safe space in our minds and invite Havi to join us there. Afterwards, Matt describes his meditation to Dr. Jo and me with tears streaming down his cheeks:

I was in the house where we stayed in Tomales Bay, in the kitchen. I saw Havi from behind, sitting in her chair at the end of the table. I could hear the waves crashing against the foundation under the cottage. The back door was open and the sea breeze was intermittently blowing through the opening. I came up beside her and bent my head next to hers. She giggled and laughed and tipped her head back, opened her mouth and took little bites out of the air. For a moment it felt so real. And then she was gone. It was the closest I felt to her since she died. And losing her again in that moment was devastating.

In my meditation, I am with Havi in the white rocking chair at home. I feel her. Her legs wrap around my pregnant belly. I massage her calves. She nuzzles into my neck. Her eyes are wet with tears. I try to wipe them, but I can't. Then she sneezes and giggles and tries to catch her breath from laughing so hard. I tuck her hair behind her ear. And before I can say goodbye, she is gone. I am not strong enough at the moment to share out loud the way Matt had.

We leave the farm on the following Sunday afternoon and head back to Phoenix to catch the red-eye home to Boston. We hold hands almost the entire drive back down from the mountains. In a few short days Matt and I had found a natural rhythm with each other and with Havi's spirit. Our visit with Dr. Jo exceeds our expectations. We have another place Havi's spirit can call home.

CHAPTER 42

Transitions

The completion of the Havi Half on the first Sunday of May starts a count-down to the departure date of Grandi and Grandadders, who will return home to Philadelphia after living for a year in Boston. We take them out to a neighborhood restaurant, sit outside on a tented patio, and order nearly everything on the menu.

As we eat, we talk about Havi. Matt and I thank them for everything they've been for us, and for Havi, and now for Kaia. I hate the fact that they are leaving Boston. We had established an easy rhythm with them, and it will be unsettling when they aren't a mile away anymore. They have become a constant source of comfort and love for Matt and me, and for Kaia; revert-ing back to a long-distance, phone-based relationship feels unsatisfying.

Havi showed us all that there is a richer, fuller way of living—one that is about being close to the people we love, valuing ritual and spirituality, grounding ourselves in the present moment. She taught us to appreciate what we do have, not to obsess over what we wish we had. My parents' return to Philadelphia feels to me like a big step backwards from where Havi had brought us. But despite the never-ending waves of my grief and my misgivings about their leaving, I also gain some clarity about what I need in the next phase of my life. I will give my one year's notice at SquashBusters.

I was handing in my resignation, but it wouldn't be effective for another whole year. Fortunately, for me, I could do this because SquashBusters isn't a typical organization. It is a real, raw, enduring com-munity whose members sustained me for nine years—the place where I found my professional voice; felt inspired daily by the hundreds of stu-dents who participated in our programs, wanting to make something of themselves and this world; and met my mentors as well as Tia—through her oldest son Edward who was one of my students, and now feels like family.

Everyone at SquashBusters, especially Greg and Rosemary, were in lockstep with us since the day of Havi's diagnosis. But I know it is time to move on, to center my life on sharing Havi's story and her essence with the world to support other families like ours. I don't know exactly what form sharing Havi with the world will take, but I know it deserves my time and attention. There are too many people in the world suffering from traumatic loss, and too few support systems and people who can hold the suffering of another for me not to try to make a difference. I want to be part of a seismic cultural shift in this country about how we talk about grief and loss and love.

So on this June morning, I take a walk in our neighborhood with Greg, who wears his Havi Half T-shirt, and I tell him that I am different now. I explain that my life's purpose has changed, that I need to figure out how to stay close to Havi's spirit and somehow honor her, and that I am committed to doing that. I tell him I need time and space to explore this new life Matt and I are creating, and that even though I still have no idea what it will look like, I know it can't be the way it is. Greg understands because he is wise, humane, and centered. He cares honestly about people. We agree that we'll spend one more year together to make sure the transition is smooth.

* * *

We filed a lawsuit against the doctors who made the mistake in Matt's Tay-Sachs screening. Our stance is that Havi didn't deserve to be born with two copies of that mutant gene, and had we known, we would have found a different way to bring her into the world. Also, we have an unshakeable conviction that what had happened to us should never happen to another family, and Matt knows enough about the internal workings of the medical system to propose practical changes to remedy this. We manage to keep most of the work regarding the lawsuit in the background of our lives, but soon Matt and I expect to be sitting for depositions with lawyers representing the doctors, and as that late June date grows closer, it begins to weigh more heavily on our minds.

The first of our two prep sessions with our own lawyers leaves Matt and me feeling empty. Afterwards, we take a long run and talk about what parts of the day were hard and painful, and what parts were empowering. By the time we get back to the car, we feel like we have our feet underneath us again. That prep session is followed two days later by nearly a full day of taped interviews of the two of us at home. The videographer had to pause recording to wipe tears from his eyes and then he thanked us for introducing him to Havi. Our lawyers plan to edit our interviews into a short video that tells Havi's story for opposing counsel. We spend five hours with them, nearly every minute of which we have tears steadily running down our faces.

We begin the day in Havi's bedroom, and I speak first. I point out the photos of Havi, one by one, and describe what is going on in each. Then Matt and I are interviewed separately. For the first time, we individually revisit every aspect of the story all at once, and on tape: Havi's birth, her slowed development, the diagnostic nightmare journey from developmental delay to the realization that she will die from Tay-Sachs, the slow and insidious loss of all her skills and strength, and eventually her death. The whole experience opens the faucet for all of our feelings and I realize yet again, but somehow more fully this time, just how much pain and sorrow we are carrying and how raw it still is. Even so, the day is a positive one because it gives us a chance to feel close to Havi, and to be her parents again. Ultimately, that's why we decided to move forward with a lawsuit. We will never get to advocate for Havi in school, to help her navigate challenges with friends, to support her through job negotiations. This lawsuit is all we have. It gives us a platform to advocate for her life.

The lawyers leave late that afternoon. It is warm outside, but the sky is gray and soon it starts to drizzle. Matt and I feel pretty wrecked so we decide to take a short walk around the neighborhood. He carries an umbrella, and even though I say I don't need it, that I don't mind getting wet, I stay close to him. I let him put his arm around me.

When we get home, the Shabbirthday preparations are in full swing. The Sibs, Kelsey, and Aunt Maggie have arrived for dinner. We scoop up Kaia and eat a delicious meal, toasting Havi multiple times and laughing and crying as we all feel her so close by.

CHAPTER 43

The "W" Word

June 16, 2021. Havi is five months gone. Kaia is almost one year old.
It is Wednesday, a Havi day, which is holy in our house. Matt and I try not
to work full days on Wednesdays. The only thing on our schedule today is
our weekly appointment with Dr. Jo. Matt and I are in the kitchen making lunch, weeks before Kaia's first birthday, when Tia bounces up the
back steps into the kitchen, dripping with sweat and flushed from a stroll
around the nearby pond with Kaia in the current heatwave. She hands a
sleeping Kaia to Matt, pours herself a glass of water, gulps it down, and
turns to face us. "You guys! She walked!"

Matt and I drop our sandwiches and stare at each other. Tia used the
W-word—*walking*. For nearly three years, that word had not belonged in
our home. It was too painful, and anyone who visited us when Havi was
alive had known not to use it to ask us if it was happening for Havi yet.

"Kaia actually *walked?*" I repeat.

I search Tia's face. Our eyes lock. "Yes," she says. "I promise."

As if on cue, Kaia starts crying in Matt's arms.

Havi. Her absence pulses through my body, in tandem with Kaia's
presence.

"Let's show Mommy and Daddy!" Tia takes Kaia back and sets her in
the middle of the kitchen floor.

"Come on, sweet girl," Matt says excitedly. "Let's see it!!"

My heartbeat quickens. A knot forms in my throat. I go to Kaia and
pull her up to standing with my sweaty palms. She grabs my hands and
clenches her tight tiny fists around my index fingers. We wait, all three of
us holding our breath. Kaia lets go of my fingers. I take a few big backward
steps. Matt crouches a few feet away, recording the scene on his phone.

"Walk to Mommy, Kaia girl," Tia urges her.

Kaia looks around. She looks at Tia. She looks at Matt. She looks at
me. And then she takes six wobbly steps toward me. With every step, my

heart explodes. I feel the presence of both of my daughters. As Kaia gets close she reaches out her hands and flops into my arms. Smiling and crying at once, I smother Kaia in kisses. Like Havi, I pray silently, please let Kaia know only our unconditional love.

"Do it again! Walk to Daddy!" Matt cheers Kaia on, crouching now.

Back and forth between us our daughter walks, taking a few steps and sitting down hard and standing up and walking again, wobbling her way from my arms to Matt's.

So. This is what it feels like to watch your child take her first steps. I get it now: the feelings of pride and melting adoration. This is the reason parents forever remember the day their child first walked. Why the W-word gets so much airtime in moms' groups and playgroups.

We had to work so hard with Havi to get her to do the smallest things. *She* had to work so hard. Now I see that with a healthy child, these skills just appear on their own, as if from some secret blueprint imprinted in her DNA. I feel a wave of remorse. *Havi*, I call out to her in my mind, *I'm so sorry we made you suffer.*

Tia takes an elated Kaia upstairs for her nap. In the quiet kitchen, Matt and I cry in each other's arms. We walk upstairs to our bedroom and collapse onto our bed. We have just been catapulted back into the world of the living: milestones and celebrations and forward progress; the deepest pride and enthusiasm and love for Kaia; and a future that suddenly looks like the one we'd imagined for Havi. We *would* get to walk alongside our daughter as she grew up.

And I'm tugged back to the world of the dead, where another version of all of those same anticipations, milestones, and missed celebrations has to sit, at an unreachable distance. They will never be experienced. That tug hurts. I cuddle up to Matt, looking for solace. In his embrace, I feel how badly he needs the same. We need arms to hold the both of us. That's why we're so lucky to have Dr. Jo, and Charlie and Blyth, and our families, I remind myself.

After a short nap, Matt and I change into our running clothes and drive to our sacred spot.

We park the car; we lace up our running shoes. Like Kaia, Matt and I are figuring out how to keep putting one foot in front of the other. "I'm so proud of Kaia. I kind of can't believe it. Can you?" I ask in wonder.

"I really can't. Footsteps!" Matt answers. "I've been waiting so long for footsteps in our house. I used to dream about them for Havi."

"So you think Kaia is totally fine?"

"What do you mean?"

I sigh. "I guess the fear doesn't go away. I still worry that something might be wrong." Matt stops. "My, Kaia is *fine*. She'll be running with us before you know it."

I laugh. I know he's right. And I decide my fear needs a way to express itself. I'm hoping it can show up as deeper love and appreciation.

When we get home, Kaia is still asleep. "She tuckered herself out with all that walking," Tia says, and hugs us both, leaving for the day. Reveling in our quiet house, I walk into Havi's room, sit in the white rocker, and write to her. I tell her about her amazing little sister who just learned to walk. I tell her that I felt her there, holding Kaia up. Just as I write that, Kaia starts to cry. It's playtime again.

Matt, Kaia, and I water Havi's blueberry bushes together. We go inside and push Kaia's pink plastic car up and down the hall. When Kaia climbs onto the little pink car's seat, she plants her feet firmly on the floor, and I remember Havi's toes, always stiff and pointed at the ground.

CHAPTER 44

Deposition Day

Matt and I intentionally choose Wednesday, June 18, for our deposition, since Wednesdays are Havi days and we want her as present as possible. Jacob drives us to our lawyer's office in downtown Boston.

Our car ride is quiet, and yet having Jacob with us gives me a sense of calm and confidence that I need. "Just be yourselves," he says a few times to break the silence. "Channel Havi," he adds.

When he pulls over to let us out at the office building, I run around to the driver's side to give him a hug and can feel his heart racing fast. He hasn't let on, but he is nervous for us. I can tell by the pitch of his voice and the red blotches on his cheeks. Our appointment is for 10:00 a.m. but we arrive two hours early so we can get settled and do some final prep with our lawyers: Rick and Laura. In order to represent us, Rick needed a partner who practiced in Massachusetts, as he was not licensed there, so through Jay, again, we found and hired Laura, who has the reputation of being the best medical malpractice lawyer in Massachusetts. The combination of Rick and Laura seems invincible. Still, I am nervous, my stomach is tight, and I have no appetite—I skipped breakfast but still make frequent trips to the bathroom.

We review our case in terms of timeline of events and the various best practices for handling a deposition. Keep your answers short and concise, make eye contact; don't yell or curse; never guess; and tell the truth. That feels straightforward enough, except maybe the part about not showing our anger. Finally, it is time to begin. The opposing attorneys enter the conference room. They shake our hands and make brief eye contact with us. As I look into their eyes, I search for their souls, wondering how they can defend this case. For the next six hours, Matt and I answer their questions firmly, concisely, and most importantly, honestly. They pepper Matt about his own knowledge of genetics, which I find insulting and irrelevant, but our lawyers reassure us afterwards that the deposition couldn't have gone better. Everything is so clear: the opposing side's error, a fatal error that is almost too obvious—which is a relief and also makes me sick.

After it is over, we walk out into the streets of downtown Boston feeling exhausted, broken, and maybe a little empowered. It is dizzying. We order an Uber back home, and once there, gather around the table with the Sibs to eat pizza and ice cream. Then we put Kaia to bed and fall fast asleep ourselves.

CHAPTER 45

Kaia Turns One

Kaia's first birthday begins at 5:50 a.m. with "Mama" and "Dada" calls to us from her bedroom. She is wide awake and ready to get moving, so we spend most of the morning watching her walk laps around her room in her beige onesie with the word "Friends" across the front, which is sized for six-to-nine-month-old babies but fits our petite one-year-old perfectly.

I open the front door and collect the mail. The lavendula is blooming; it's full of brilliant purple flowers and wraps all the way around the house.

Erin surprises Kaia with a strawberry-frosted donut, which they feed to each other until most of the donut ends up on the floor. Leah sends photos of Havi and Kaia together on the day Kaia is born, and by mid-morning, Kaia discovers the wrapped presents from all her aunts and uncles, grandparents, and her cousins Ayla and Hannah stacked in a pile on the living room floor. She sits right down and starts ripping them open. By evening, we gather to celebrate Kaia with cake and more presents with her grandparents, all her aunts and uncles, Tia and her family, and Charlie and Blyth. Her two vacuum cleaners—one from Charlie and Blyth and one from Aunt Leah and Uncle Mike—are Kaia's favorite gifts, which makes Matt very proud, as he is known to appreciate a good vacuum session. Kaia stands a little taller in her yellow summer dress, cheeks flushed from playing out in the sun, and we smother her with kisses before putting her to bed.

Matt and I snuggle in bed. Then he turns to me. "We fucked up for Havi's first birthday. Barely celebrated. I feel like we missed that whole first year caught up in all the day-to-day bullshit."

"We couldn't have known. I'd do anything to go back," I reply.

"Yeah, same. I'm hoping we did this one right by Kaia. She deserves every ounce of love and more."

* * *

On a very rainy Friday in July, I meet Blyth at a restaurant for lunch. As I arrive, the rain turns into a downpour, so before I exit the car, I zip my rain jacket and pull my hood up, then make a dash for the covered entrance to the dining room. Luckily, I only have to wait for a minute until I see Blyth walking toward me, holding an umbrella. Immediately, my body relaxes and I smile. I always feel safe and inspired with Blyth, and this is to be our first one-to-one lunch date. We have spent a lot of time together before, but always as a group of four, with Matt and Charlie. This time it is just the two of us because we've made plans to talk about Courageous Parents Network (CPN), Blyth's nonprofit organization, and the ways in which my own exploration of what would come next in my life might intersect with Blyth's work.

Havi feels very present for me as Blyth and I make our way to our table, and I'm aware of the fact that it is she who brought me to Blyth. I try not to think too much about what that actually means, but just appreciate that she brought me my beautiful new mentor and friend.

We each order a salad and split a tuna melt. She orders a peppermint tea which seems to fit with the wet weather and I do the same. Our conversation flows naturally, as it always has. She tells me the stories of some of the incredible people she's met who have also endured the loss of a child and describes the memoir manuscripts of some aspiring authors who have stories for the world. Blyth also tells me about some of the important work CPN is doing to make families feel less alone and invites me to become involved—she even commits to putting things in my path to which I could choose to invest time and energy, or not. No pressure either way.

We top off our two-hour lunch with cookies for dessert and I confess my tendency to pass up opportunities that come my way. I seem to have fallen into a pattern of not taking things to the next level, I tell her. That was true in soccer, in graduate school, and in my career—and it feels true now. In soccer, I could have scored more goals, possibly even played professionally after college; for graduate school, I applied and was waitlisted at my dream school but then never advocated to get off the waitlist; and professionally, I was often curious about whether I could expand my scope of influence beyond my local community. Simply curious. Now, I wonder, out loud for the first time, where this hesitancy comes from.

Blyth offers her perspective: "Maybe you haven't wanted your full light to shine. Maybe you don't realize how big your light can be." Maybe. No one has ever put it that way to me before. I feel empowered.

The rain stops just as it is time to go home. I need to hurry because it is Friday, after all, and soon to be the Shabbirthday hour. When I get back in my car, I find that I have twenty minutes left of an *On Being* podcast—Krista Tippett interviewing Joanna Macy, a translator of Rilke and a Buddhist philosopher of ecology.

Macy's voice comes through the car speakers: "Because when things are this unstable, a person's determination, how they choose to invest their energy, and their heart-mind can have much more effect on the larger picture than we're accustomed to think."

I take this as validation that I should let my full light shine, as Blyth suggested. If I am here on earth without Havi, then I owe it to both of us to try to have an effect on the world beyond my family and my own community. I am fully aware of all the privilege I have, though Havi's life and death put it into an even greater focus. I ache for families who lose a child and have to return to work three days later; for families who don't have any support system at all to help take care of their child(ren); for those who can't escape to the beach or the mountains to get some air when they felt like they were suffocating; for couples in marriages that won't last.

I am learning how to stay in close contact with my own pain, and how that deepens my understanding of suffering and enhances my ability to be there for others who are also suffering. And maybe, by being there for others who endure traumatic loss—or, frankly, any meaningful loss—I can find ways back to Havi. In some form or another, I will share her essence with the world. This much I know.

As I pull up our driveway, I feel both wounded and grateful. I park the car, look up at Havi and Kaia's windows, take a long, deep breath, and walk through the front door of our beautiful, love-filled, and broken home.

CHAPTER 46

The Six-Month Mark

"I don't want it to be six months. It's too long." Matt turns toward me with tears in his eyes.

I swallow hard, "I know. I hate it."

Matt and I sit next to each other on the couch in Havi's room, our legs touching. It is July 20 at 9:04 a.m.—six months from the moment Havi took her last breath in my arms.

We stare at the long string of photos of her that hang on her bedroom wall.

Where are you? I plead with her, silently. *Can you visit us soon?*

Anguish moves through my body in waves and pulses. It sits in my throat and wells in my eyes. It radiates along my skin in prickly tingles and fills my chest with heaviness. My arm extends toward her simple white dresser and I reach for her pajama drawer, the bottom right drawer that I used to open thoughtlessly so many times, and pull on the handle. Her pastel-striped onesie with a fuzzy unicorn across the chest sits on top of the pile of her carefully folded clothes. I bring it to my face and bury my head in it, sobbing.

Matt puts his hand on my leg. I remove it. "Please don't. I'm with Havi now," I whisper.

My eyes stay tightly shut, soaking her pajamas with my tears. My mind is fuzzy and I stop feeling my body on the couch. I am with Havi, in the white rocking chair that still sits in its spot across the room. The lights are off, the shade is drawn. I can see her beautiful features in the soft light that sneaks through the small crack at the bottom of the shade. Her legs wrap around my waist, and her head nestles into my neck just below where my jawbone makes that sharp turn. My left hand rests on her left cheek, and my right hand supports her bottom. I start to hum our song: "Have I told you lately that I love you?"

We fall back into our nighttime routine so naturally. And then she is gone.

Have I imagined her presence? Or has she actually visited my heart-mind? It's a distinction worth pondering. Because what is imagination, if not a self-created reality? And why is that any more or less real than any other moment in time?

I open my eyes and wipe them with the back of my hand. I refold her now-damp-with-tears unicorn onesie, open the drawer, and place it back in its spot, on top of her other clothes. I close the drawer.

It is the first time I have opened any of her drawers since the day she died six months ago. I don't think I'm avoiding pain. I am able to stare pain right in the eyes. So then, why is seeing her clothing in the dresser drawer different from sitting in the car without her car seat, or staring at the photos we've got of her all over our home, or watching Kaia use the baby spoons we bought for Havi when she transitioned from breastmilk to solids? What am I so afraid I'll find in, or feel from her pajamas? Amid this odyssey of thoughts, a profound realization emerges. Opening the drawer reveals a wellspring, a depth of feeling that brings me even closer to Havi. Deep in that drawer lives an alchemy of pain and beauty, and it needs a stir. And giving it that stir deepens me.

For a moment, I am close to her. Not because any part of me believes that she is somehow still in those pajamas, but because I let myself feel.

CHAPTER 47

Soaking Wet

One Wednesday morning in early August, on a cool day with overcast skies, Matt and I clear our calendars, leave Kaia with Aunt Leah, and slip out of the house by 7:15 a.m. We drive south for thirty minutes, winding through the outskirts of Boston and into the suburbs, to the Skyline Trail that starts in Quincy. A couple of kids shoot hoops on a court across the street from the parking lot; otherwise, it is quiet. We lace up our trail shoes, pull on our backpacks, which hold water bottles and a few nutrition bars and cross the pavement to the woods, where we can lose ourselves in the green earth. Over the next fifteen miles of classic New England trails, our only company is the rich canopy of trees and plants—and, as it turns out, quite a few mosquitos.

This is how all Wednesday mornings should start. *Live full!* For most of the days of Havi's short life, she urged us out into the natural world with bright eyes chasing the light and her little mouth opening to swallow the taste of the wind. That's how she taught us we're part of something bigger than our fragile bodies, and let us know that after she left, we'd be able to find her in the greater forces of the earth.

As we bob and weave over the rocky terrain of the tree-lined trail we pay close attention to our steps, keeping our eyes pointed down most of the way. The motion of my shoes sliding forward and back, over and around the gray stones, becomes meditative. The surrounding forest blurs in my peripheral vision, but I feel its presence hum around me.

From the day of Havi's diagnosis to the day of her death, I paid closer attention to everything around me than before. I kept my eyes on the only thing that mattered, and let the rest of the world blur and then fade to the periphery. And you know what I missed? Nothing. Because paying attention to the things that matter is the only thing that matters—family, nature, long meals, slow dancing, laughter.

Yet, our noisy world is confusing and distracting and celebrates superficiality over authenticity. So we get lost—in comparisons of whose house is nicer, who gets the better promotion, how incredible that family's trip to Hawaii looks in their pictures on Instagram. Even after holding Havi through seizures and then lying there trembling as she took her last breath on my chest in our bed, I still worry about whether I stack up or not. I still get insecure about the promotions I notice other people posting on their LinkedIn profiles—promotions that I am not getting. I still wonder whether I'm achieving enough. The tug of the world of the living takes its toll, and so does the world of the privileged, where ambition and ego seem to get the better of us if we aren't paying close attention. If we don't welcome the bigger world.

On this Wednesday morning in August, getting to the woods helps. We quickly reach the midpoint, the top of the steepest climb, which is literally a stairway made of rock straight up the side of the Great Blue Hill. I turn around to look back for Matt. I hear him before I see him— *squoosh, squoosh, squoosh*—he is soaked with sweat, right down to his shoes. Suddenly I remember him throwing me into the pool at a barbeque before we were dating. On that day, ten years ago, I was quick to grab his arm as he launched me toward the water so that he fell in too, and we both ended up soaking wet. I'd been annoyed, but excited. It was the first time I thought maybe we'd date. Now, I feel a rush of gratitude on the trail for him having thrown me into the pool that day, despite the fact that it led to us suffering together the worst loss imaginable.

"How are you?" I call out. It is a bit of an empty question, though. I know the answer from his slowing pace, heavy breathing, and pale-white face.

"Great!" he lies, looking just as he did when pulling himself up from that swimming pool.

So we slow down to share an energy bar and then turn to head back down the trail for the second leg, both smiling, aching, and wet: a small moment of ecstasy. We are in sync with the woods and each other, the rhythm and sound of our steps part of nature's thrum. That's why we had gone for a run: for that feeling, for being reminded that we too are part of something greater. In the midst of that realization, I feel Havi *just* a little bit closer, even if my two feet are still in the world of the living. Havi's world, the world of the dead, seems to come most alive for me in the woods. We know this lesson. Getting into nature helps. Nature is quiet, nonjudgmental, and demands nothing from us, yet also invites us to breathe and connect to a universe that is much bigger than ourselves.

During the final miles back to the car, my legs begin to ache, but then the gift of a flat stretch of trail relieves me. Soon we hit another steep slope, and slow to a walk or maybe climb hand-over-hand. The run we chose is painful, hard, and grueling, and I'm grateful for all of it.

I think a lot of people misunderstand gratitude. We need to feel grateful *and* feel pain. That's the only way for hearts to stretch and grow. Gratitude doesn't minimize pain. Gratitude enhances beauty, and pain always sits right alongside beauty. Sometimes beauty is jagged and sharp and unforgiving, like a rocky East Coast trail.

Back in the car, heading home, Matt desperately needs to rehydrate, so we pull over at the first corner store we find and pick up Coke, Gatorade, and a bottle of water. First the ecstasy, then the corner store. All before noon on a Wednesday in August.

* * *

Dear Peanut,

I turned thirty-nine today, and it was my first birthday since you died. Our celebrations are different now.

Life feels distant and strange; fogged over in the haze of disbelief and shattered dreams. I wander through the house looking at the hundreds of photos of you, of us, that are strung up on the walls or in frames on mantles, shelves, and windowsills. Was that our life? It looks like our hearts were fuller then, in the months before your diagnosis, and even more in the months afterward. And what am I doing now? I don't know.

Your brief existence on this earth transformed me. You made me see the spirit and the soul as part of a larger force. You yanked me out of the rut of silly societal expectations and laid the important questions, the good questions, the best questions, right in front of me. You stripped away the distractions and shut out the noise so I could hear the sounds of the earth and my own heartbeat. We lived in the bubble with you, somewhere in between the world of the living and the world of the dead. We lived in liminal space. We are doing everything we can to stay there, but it's a hard place to exist without you in it.

I am looking for a new job. It was time to leave my company, even though they have been wonderful to me, and to us, and to figure out where work fits into the larger framework of my life. I'm not sure where I'll land, but I need to look elsewhere.

Kaia wandered into your room yesterday afternoon while your mom and I were in there—it was a Wednesday, a Havi day. She climbed the three stairs from the main floor quickly, using her hands and feet, and tottered down the hall in a stumble-run. Her existence is full of jiggling energy, like what I would imagine an electron would be like if it were blown-up to toddler size. She found your photo on your rocker, the one that shows you lying on a blanket with your straw-colored hair in small curls against the gray fabric. You are smiling and your eyes are twinkling—they look so alive, even in the photo, which I've stared at so many times. Kaia picked the photo up with her two little hands and walked a few steps across the room with her back to Mom and me. She was babbling—talking with you in some secret sister language. And then she brought the photo to her face and kissed it twice, with big beautiful, exaggerated, cartoon-like kisses. "Mwwaah! Mwwaah!"

We all love you.

Dad

CHAPTER 48

To Life

I am reading John O'Donohue again, and Matt is finishing *Harry Potter*. He puts his kindle down and turns to my side of the bed. "Are you sure you are ready? It's going to be hardest on you, on your body."

"Yes. I am. I want Kaia to have a living sibling."

"And we aren't going to tell anyone? Still?"

"Yeah, I think we should hold off until we have a better sense of how everything is going to turn out. Too much loss already. I don't want to bring anyone else into this yet."

"Okay, baby. Then let's start, as the nurse said we can, next week. Based on your cycle.

Matt pulls me close and kisses my cheek. "I love you."

We decided, some months earlier, to pursue IVF so we could continue to grow our family. We know now that if we are to conceive naturally, there is a twenty-five percent chance of having another child with Tay-Sachs. The decision for IVF is not an easy one to make, but we eventually arrive there because it gives us reassurance that we could have a healthy child. We want Kaia to have a living sibling, and we want more of both Havi and Kaia in this world. After all, siblings are the most genetically similar human beings on earth.

Over these summer months I go to all the necessary appointments: ultrasounds, blood draws, and various screening tests required for insurance approval. Then come all the hormone injections, which we do at home. Matt gets up early to prepare my needles and inject them into me and is always there when I need an ice pack afterward. He endures my mood swings and reassures me whenever I feel unsure about the process.

* * *

My egg retrieval takes place on Havi's memorial weekend. I take this as a sign that she approves of our decision to expand our family. We hold Havi's memorial service on Labor Day weekend because it's Havi's birthday and our wedding anniversary. We invite a large group of friends and family, hoping that by September Covid would be relatively under control and people could travel safely. Now, though, the Delta variant hits and some of our family members can't make the trip. Still, hundreds of people come to honor Havi's life. We gather in a grassy field behind an old country-inn turned restaurant in Sherborn, Massachusetts. We had spent a handful of spring days with Havi on trails in the Sherborn woods and at a pond nearby. There is familiarity and safety in this space, and it has Havi's essence all over it.

Our posse transforms the space inside into a journey through the essence of Havi—photos line the restaurant walls and tables are set with all of Havi's albums, handmade blankets, and her "scents" (shampoo, body lotion, laundry detergent, etc.) all captured in little glass jars. A television in the corner plays Havi's giggle video, compiled by Leah, on repeat. Everyone wears lavender and eats Havi's favorite foods: cheesy eggs, blueberry pancakes, avocados, and smoothies. Charlie and Blyth open the service, followed by prayers, poems, and shared memories that bring us all from tears to laughter and back again. The band that played at Havi's second birthday makes a special trip to play for Havi again. The ceremony ends with Andrea singing a soul-shaking version of "For Good" from the musical *Wicked*. And then we dance, to all of Havi's favorite songs with Kaia sitting atop Matt's shoulders encircled by our closest people, her arms waving up in the air.

Havi's posse yet again elevates her presence in all our lives and undoubtedly leaves a Havi print on the hearts of everyone who attends. Matt and I hug and thank everyone who shows up for us. Show up for people. On big and small days. It always matters.

By the time everyone clears out, the posse has cleaned everything up and packed the cars. Matt and I hold hands and walk through the restaurant out to the front parking lot where Hav's posse waits. We drive home listening to "You Should Be Here" on repeat.

CHAPTER 49

The Last Supper

Soon the high from Havi's memorial service fades and the all-too-familiar pain returns. As the world slowly reopens from the pandemic, tugs of prepandemic life begin to pull on our fragile bubble. On September 24, we host what we call "our last supper." It is the last dinner we have together with all of the Sibs as Boston residents. Jacob and Erin are moving to Nashville for a work opportunity that they can't pass up. Mike's law firm returns to in-office work as the Texas courts reopen, and Leah's speech and language lab also reopens soon, so they will be heading back to Dallas.

After Matt and I tuck Kaia into bed we gather in the kitchen. We sit down to eat at the round table that Ali's husband, Greg, spent the last year building. It is a beautiful table, handmade from wood that comes from fallen trees pulled from Lake Geneva, just a few blocks from their home. Greg built it in his garage, quietly working all through the winter. He inlayed a small letter "H," for Havi, on the underside. When we carried it into the kitchen last week, we rotated the "H" to align with the place where Havi used to sit. Something about the round table made our posse feel even closer. We eat slowly and quietly. No one knows what to say; too much has happened. Then Matt pulls out his phone and reads aloud a note he started to write a few days before in anticipation of their departure:

> Blyth told Myra and me the other day that what we—all of us—have created and experienced in the last two years will be with us forever. I know that it has changed us all, deeply. In a way, Havi made life seem so simple. She made it profoundly easy to live in congruence with the most important values and to stay surrounded by only the people who really matter. You guys arrived here and joined your arms together

to surround us with safety and strength. I know you say that it was the only option, but I know that it didn't have to be that way. You have taught me so much about myself and maybe, more importantly, about who I ultimately want to be.

With tears in everyone's eyes, we stand up and give each other big, long hugs. It feels like we could stay that way forever, but suddenly Kaia's loud, piercing cry rises from her bedroom. She has other plans. Like Havi, not the best sleeper. "Can I go in?" Erin pleads.

"Can I go, too?" Leah adds.

We are sleep-training Kaia, which they know. "I guess tonight can be an exception," I say with a smile.

"I'll scoop the ice cream tonight," Matt says.

"I'm on dishes," Jacob said.

"Great, I'll take a seat in my favorite chair," Mike replies.

Our families and Havi's entire posse near and far, taught us what is truly the greatest lesson of all: activate people who make you feel good, and stay away from those who don't. Relationships change inherently after an experience like ours. It's inevitable that some people will be better able than others to accept who you've become. For Matt and me, the people who embrace how we have changed and how Havi has forever marked us, and who help us to hold her with us, are the people worth our time and energy. Those who can't, for whatever reason, integrate and honor Havi, at least for now, we do not accommodate. It just hurts too much.

CHAPTER 50

Weighty Matters

Soon it is October, a month already since Havi's memorial service. The leaves are changing from greens to yellows and oranges and reds, and the mornings and evenings have gotten a bit too cool to wear shorts and a t-shirt. I feel out of sorts and spend a lot of time thinking about what *out of sorts* actually means.

Charlie and Blyth join us for dinner a few nights before my scheduled embryo transfer. Being with them continues to feel so right, especially on the cusp of a hopeful pregnancy. They drink too much and we all laugh a lot. We talk about what Blyth and Charlie do to stay close to Cameron, how their work with the Courageous Parents Network sometimes does and sometimes doesn't make them feel close to her. We talk about money, and our families, how to make sure our inner selves see us the way we ought to be seen, and how even the most remarkable people have a hard time quieting the noise of this crazy world of ambition and expectations and superficial markers of success. I decide I will continue to breathe deeply and draw Havi in every time I move too close to one of those danger zones of toxic comparisons

Since I resigned from my job with a year's notice, my role as chief program and strategy officer is now open to the outside world. We post the job description and, slowly, résumés start coming in. I am hopeful that we'll find someone great so that I can devote my time to writing a book about Havi and our life. That's what feels right, at least in the moment.

Also, we settle the lawsuit, and share this news with Charlie and Blyth. We decide against waiting for years to present our case to a jury because, due to Covid, the courts are backed up significantly. As part of the settlement, the hospital agrees to change the test ordering system to prevent this error from ever happening to another family. We're also allowed to share our full story. This feels important. To not hide. To begin our journey to supporting other families who are grieving. We don't know how exactly, but we know that sharing Havi's story is where we'll start.

* * *

Finally, we reach the moment of the embryo transfer, the final stage of a long, cumbersome process. So, one morning just before Halloween, Matt and I head back to Brigham and Women's Hospital for another monumental life experience. Matt hasn't been back there regularly like I have over these past six months, so it triggers him to be there again, and I watch his whole body tense up as we walk through the front doors of the building at 75 Francis.

When we enter the elevator, his face turns pale. "I hate this place. I can't be in here."

"Seriously, Em, how do you think I feel? I am here basically every day. I kind of need you right now."

"I am just telling you how I feel."

His relationship with this hospital is more fraught than mine. It's where he trained to become a doctor. Matt's work at Brigham and Women's was what brought us to Boston in the first place, and where I gave birth to Havi, and to Kaia. I can understand why he has a hard time knowing how to feel in this space. And yet, I need him to be okay.

The embryo transfer procedure itself takes fewer than five minutes. Afterwards, we return home to Kaia, who has spent the morning with Tia. It is hard for me to process the immensity of what has just happened.

Later that day, we take Kaia to Tia's house to celebrate La Dia de los Muertos together. Tia makes an altar with beautiful photographs and tributes to all the people she has lost. There are lots of older people— grandparents, aunts, uncles. And then there is Havi. Our precious toddler looks larger than life on the altar, where Tia placed a framed photo of Havi that Leah gifted to her. Havi's mouth is open wide and her eyes are smiling brighter than I even remember they could.

It is customary on La Dia de los Muertos to make an offering of the foods that your family's beloved dead loved the most, so Tia sets a bowl of blueberries and Havi's wafer crackers out on the altar along with fresh, sliced avocado. Tia's husband, Fabian, prepares a blueberry smoothie and we toast Havi as one combined family. I am caught someplace between feeling grateful and nauseous, proud, and heartbroken—I try to say thank you to Tia and her family, but only tears come out. I don't want my daughter on an altar on the Day of the Dead. I want her to be here on earth, with us and with her sister and her aunts and uncles and grandparents.

* * *

Then Halloween arrives and, suddenly, there are too many weighty things flying around us. My Zadie—my grandfather and Havi and Kaia's great-grandfather—hasn't been doing well the past few weeks and comes down with a urinary tract infection. He receives treatment and fluids at home and my mom is hopeful that maybe he has turned a corner. But on the night after Halloween, as Matt and Kaia and I sit down to dinner, my phone rings. It is my dad. He tells us that Zadie died. He dies just six weeks before his 101st birthday.

We all drive down to Philadelphia so we can be together and take care of my mom. When we pull up to 105 Rolling Road, my childhood home, Matt and I both exhale deeply. It always feels good to be with my parents, and this time the Sibs are here, too. We jump out of the car, scoop Kaia out of her car seat, and run up the driveway. The warmest embraces await.

I need everyone. The embryo transfer hasn't worked, and I am not pregnant. In a few days I will speak to the doctor to learn more about what happened and what the plan will be moving forward. But for now, we are surrounded by love and warmth and share memories of my grandfather which remind us of just how long and rich life can be.

It feels so right for us to be back together again. Returning to Boston will be hard, but Matt and I are learning to be gentler with ourselves during these transitions.

* * *

Friday, November 19, 2021

Dear Peanut,

Earlier this week I dreamt about you. It was the first dream where you've visited me since a week or so after you died. I was standing in the living room of a cabin on a lake. You were lying on the couch, with your head on a pillow, your golden curls radiating out across the pillow's surface. I was looking down at you; you smiled your biggest open-mouthed smile and moved your head back and forth—I could hear your amazing giggle starting to form somewhere deep inside your belly.

Later that day, Mom was in the passenger seat and I was driving, my eyes wet with tears as we waited at the red light. It was a bright and beautiful day; the sky was a sharp blue and while the sun was strong, it was only in the low 30s outside. Every day I get up, I do the things I need to do, and I make it to dinner and then to bed. And every day I get further and further from the days when I could walk into your room and scoop you up. I turned to Mom and said, "I want to go back, I know that I can't, but I want to so badly." Maybe that's what dreams are for—a brief moment to go back.

A lot of people have been telling us that we're so resilient, as if we've been able to bounce back, snap back into some semblance of normal, or at least into some semblance of life before Tay-Sachs. Mom said that she likes the word "stamina" better than "resilience." Stamina is the Latin word meaning "life threads spun by the fates." It shares the same root with "stamen," the part of the flower that produces pollen. Pollen is able to fly, levitate, phase through solid objects, and carry objects heavier than itself. Whoa. So yeah, I like "stamina" a lot better too.

I love you, sweet girl. Forever and beyond.

Dad

* * *

On Thanksgiving weekend, Matt parks the stroller on the side of the Minuteman Path in Lincoln, a thirty-minute drive northwest from our house, and we follow Kaia around as she scales rocks and hides behind trees, coaxing us into variations of hide-and-seek and tag. The fifty-degree weather means the country path is heavily trafficked. As each of the runners and walkers pass us, Kaia greets them with a wave and, "Bye-bye." At only twenty pounds and standing knee-high, Kaia makes her presence known to this world.

She is beautiful with big brown eyes and long eyelashes, the cutest little ears, and Matt's skin tone—olive and easily tanned. And she has a beautiful smile with a whole mouthful of teeth. Her hair is light brown, although sometimes in the light we notice a hint of red. Havi's was that way too. It is another special feature the two of them share.

And Kaia is the boss! She knows what she wants and what she doesn't, and she's mastered the art of "No, no, no," accompanied by a wagging finger. She takes full advantage of her days. One morning, Matt brings her into our bed at 4:30 a.m., hoping she'll snooze a bit longer. Instead, she sits on his head and starts laughing and exclaiming, "Da Da Daaad." She is up, and therefore so are we. She hates to sit still. In fact, we try to watch a movie with her and after ninety seconds she promptly slides off the couch, walks to the stairs, and crawls up them until she is suddenly out of sight. We get the message and pause the movie.

She loves to make a mess and then clean it all up. After a few Cheerios, a couple bites of mac 'n cheese, or spoonfuls of applesauce, she takes great pleasure in sharing her food with the floor, the rug, and the chairs. Then, in an instant, she's off to grab a piece of paper towel to wipe it all up, and she finishes the job with a satisfied, "Dun dun," wiping her hands against each other.

Kaia loves to explore and she takes her time to study things. She has just about figured out how to open our cabinets with the magnetic lock designed to prevent toddlers from opening them! She loves to give kisses, and sometimes in the morning the three of us have "kiss trains." Matt wraps his arms around Kaia and me, and kisses Kaia on the cheek, then she kisses me, and I kiss Matt. I kiss him double for Havi girl.

Back on the Minuteman Path, Kaia yawns a few big, long ones, and follows it up with some eye-rubbing, so we know it is time for her to take a stroller nap. Matt and I walk for a few hours along the path, trying to hold onto the both/and of our first Thanksgiving without Havi and the wonder of celebrating with Kaia. Being outside helps make space for all of our feelings.

We drive to Tia's after our long walk. Matt and I both want to be wrapped in Tia's love and warmth and know she'll honor the heaviness of the day with us. Every wall in her home has a photo of Havi and Kaia on it, and we clink our wine glasses in Havi's honor and chase Kaia up and down the stairs until it is time to go home.

Then Matt and Kaia and I drive home and eat cereal with extra blueberries for Thanksgiving dinner.

CHAPTER 51

The Other Havi

December 14, 2021. Havi has been gone eleven months. Kaia is eighteen months old.

"What's your grief doing?" Dr. Jo starts every call with the same question. I never feel prepared to fully answer it. *What is my grief doing?* I ask myself.

On today's call, when Dr. Jo asks me that question, I say, "I really don't know. But I do know I'm holding a positive pregnancy test in my hand. So there's that."

We did a second embryo transfer a few days earlier. That morning, before speaking with Dr. Jo, I had a blood test which confirmed a very early pregnancy. I can't quite believe it's true. Although my emotions are complicated by the first failed transfer and the fear of another one, I have a feeling that this is a viable pregnancy, and I'm thrilled.

"Okay, this is the best, best, best," Dr. Jo says, not hiding her elation. "Incredible. And of course, this baby won't have known Havi. And that will always hurt." I'm moved by Dr. Jo's response. I am glad she says what I've been thinking and feeling. Naming it helps. When something is named, it moves from the unconscious to the conscious mind. I can work with it there.

We spend the rest of the call preparing for Diagnosis Day, three days from now: the first anniversary of Havi's terminal diagnosis, the day that started the clock on the thirteen months—December 17, 2019 to January 20, 2021—from Havi's diagnosis to her death. We'll be commemorating the first anniversary of Havi's passing, a milestone that no parent should experience.

* * *

On December 17, Diagnosis Day, I leave work early to spend the afternoon with Kaia. It's fifty-nine degrees outside. The whole week has been beautiful and warm. The magnolia tree down the street, in a state of arboreal confusion, has even started to bloom.

With Kaia in her car seat, I drive to Rosenfeld's Bakery in Newton to pick up challah for tonight's Shabbirthday. With the loaf's sweet fragrance filling the car, I Google nearby parks. A few minutes later, we pull in to a park we've never visited before.

Kaia and I walk across the basketball court toward the playground. She's wearing the pink Patagonia jacket that used to be Havi's, and Havi's purple pants with yellow butterflies on them, and Havi's purple shoes. As we approach the play structures, Kaia points to a dog tied to the playground fence and tries her best to bark, making a high-pitched sound that falls somewhere between a chirp and a woof, sounding something like "churf."

Kaia pulls me across the playground to the dog, a medium-sized Wheaton-poodle mix, golden brown with a soft fluffy coat, wearing a Chanukah scarf, which I find endearing. Kaia pets him, cooing at him, looking adorable next to him, since he's twice her size. I relax and let the warm sun blanket my face. It's Diagnosis Day. I'm being gentle with myself.

"Havi, Havi!" I hear someone shout.

What? Am I losing my mind?

An older woman walks toward us purposefully, a squirming baby under her arm and a skinny, blonde, curly-haired, blue-eyed little girl walking next to her.

"Is this your dog? Is it okay that we pet him?" I ask nervously.

"Of course!" she says. "Most perfect dog on the planet. His name is Ogie."

"I'm Myra. This is Kaia. What are the children's names? I thought I heard you say..."

"I'm Sarina. This is my grandson, Parker." She sets the baby boy down, takes the hand of the little girl. "And this is Havi."

My heart drops. My knees buckle.

"My daughter's name is Havi." I'm struggling to speak. "I've never heard her name anywhere. Ever."

"From *Chava* in Hebrew?" she asks.

"Yes, exactly. You too?"

"Yes," she says. "I can't believe you said her name correctly. Most people mispronounce it so it sounds like 'gave.' How old is your Havi?"

I'm silent for a long moment. "She, um...she actually passed away earlier this year."

"Oh." Her hand flies to her heart. "I am so sorry."

"No, no. It's okay. I can't believe we came here today. That we met you here. That we met...Havi."

Parker and Havi run off, Kaia right behind them.

"I'm so sorry," she keeps saying. "It's okay," I keep answering.

I explain that Havi had Tay-Sachs disease. I give Sarina the three lines on her life: Wrong test ordered. Tay-Sachs diagnosis. A tragic and treasured life.

We stand together in silence. "Kaia is beautiful," she says finally.

Our time together is interrupted by the kids, who start running in different directions. Kaia has found the swings. I push her back and forth, back and forth, in a state of disbelief.

Sarina joins us. I like her. She feels warm and soft.

"I can't believe this," I say. "Today is two years since we found out our Havi had Tay-Sachs. That's why I'm here."

"It's *beshert*," Sarina says, and it makes me feel even closer to her, that she's using the Yiddish word for destiny or preordained.

"Yes," I say. "It is."

"Do you want to join us for Shabbat dinner? You and your husband and Kaia?"

"Oh that's so nice of you. Tonight we can't. But another time, yes. We'd love that." And then we're both crying and hugging each other.

There's so much more to say, but we don't have the time. Sarina and I exchange phone numbers and hug our final goodbye. I chase Kaia around the playground for a while as she blows kisses and waves to everyone. I'm crying and fighting back gallons of tears, at the same time wondering if what I just experienced could possibly have been real.

Another Havi? On December 17, 2021?

Kaia and I get back in the car. I sob the whole way home. I hate crying like this in front of Kaia so I turn on Dan Zanes' "All Around the Kitchen" to drown myself out. Sarina's Havi had such big eyes, like our Havi's. Her hair is blonde and curly, like our Havi's. Would our Havi have walked like this Havi? Would she have ruled the playground the way her namesake did? Would our Havi have taken care of Kaia the way the other Havi looked after Parker?

While I drive, I glance up at the moon. I swear I see Havi there. "Come home?" I cry. "Please?"

"I'm with you, Mom," Havi answers. "Don't you know?"

CHAPTER 52

Holidays

Once again, we find ourselves in holiday season, entering the time of year that we know is particularly painful. While the rest of the world celebrates frivolously in anticipation of the New Year, we try to get through a period of time that reminds us of all the most painful things.

What feels the most painful is the contrast between what other people seem to be doing and feeling and what is happening in our home. Or maybe it has nothing at all to do with the outside world.

During these difficult weeks, Kaia climbs on the pink chair in the corner of the kitchen and points to a cluster of photos from our Havimoon. She thinks Havi is her. She points and says, "Kai-Kai, Kai-Kai," and then taps her chest with her finger. The first time I see her do this, it takes my breath away. I don't correct her. I want Kaia to know that she has a sister—a sister who'd had beautiful adventures that we can tell her about, a sister who loves Kaia even though Kaia can't see her.

And I like the fact that Kaia assumes all of these photographed moments include her, and that when she looks at Havi, she points to herself. It makes me hope that as she gets older and understands how deep and enduring a sister's bond is, she'll continue to see the two of them as forever connected.

On Christmas Day, I take a nap in Havi's bedroom after I refill her jars with shampoo, body wash, and her lotion. I doze off while I breathe in her essence, turning my cheek toward where hers would be on the pillow as I try to remember what her soft cheeks feel like against mine.

December 31, 2021

Sweetest girl, Sweetest Little Pea, Peanut—

"No one ever told me that grief felt so like fear. Perhaps, more strictly, like suspense. Or like waiting; just hanging about, waiting for something to happen." (C.S. Lewis, *A Grief Observed*)

Time has hurtled us forward and we're here at the end of the year—the last year we had you with us physically on this earth. I'm not happy about New Year's arrival, for every day lived without you is one day further away from having you in our arms. I feel the one-year anniversary of your death looming and I'm afraid of it. My mind is caught in a fog of disbelief. I'm afraid of being leveled by the intensity of revisited emotions, of the summoning of visceral memories of your last weeks, days, and breaths with us. But I'm also afraid that I won't feel the pain deeply or fully enough. I don't want to be numb, not even if it's just a little bit around the edges. I don't want to be on the other side of this first year without you either. A single day without you is too long; a year feels impossible. With time has come the forced changes in how we talk about you, how we introduce you. We've decided that the phrase we'll use from now on will be, "My daughter died last year." There is more distance there, more space for people to keep the rawness, the depth, the intensity of that fact at arm's length, so they're more comfortable with the idea. But even trying to form those words in my mouth feels bitter and hollow. Last year. There is a deeply painful shift in that.

I woke up in the middle of the night wondering whether I should have fought for you more. Should we have pursued experimental medicines, or tried to initiate trials of untested and unproven therapies? Should we have gotten you a feeding tube? I know you didn't want any of that, but sometimes I still wonder. And then today, on my golf-course run, I realized that the way you lived was your way—that you were a hero for not fighting and for instead living. Maybe you understood acceptance in the way it should be understood.

Love you,

Dad

* * *

On New Year's Eve, I sit for a while in Havi's room, my hair wet from the shower, staring out the window, wondering if the sun will ever reappear. I know it will, but not this day.

Usually writing helps make me feel better, but for some reason, it is not helping now. I wish I could just talk to Havi, and not through my journal. I want to give her a hug and a kiss and have a little goodnight snuggle before the New Year. I am feeling sorry for myself, but maybe that is okay.

Kaia is busy: running all over the house, jumping on furniture, coloring in her downstairs "classroom," picking out her own clothes, trying to put her shoes on, and chit-chatting all the while. At this point she doesn't quite have complete words, but she's already a very effective communicator. She can say the beginning of most words and gets her point across easily. She has clearly established herself as the boss around our house, and Matt and I know that Havi would have loved everything about her.

I know that this will be a year of great change because I will give birth to my third child (and my first son). How? How to be? How can I be? A new mother? A bereaved mother? Be open to all of my feelings, I tell myself. Treat yourself gently. I think about origami. Explicitly beautiful and intricate. Implicitly delicate and complicated. Strong in its contiguous structure. Sitting in Havi's room, it is impossible to not feel like I am drowning in swirling waves of the most polarized emotions. It is in these moments that I see, feel, hear, and sense the details of life in hyper-color. Anguish and joy do not oppose, they amplify. As I anticipate brand new life, I am embraced by the thin veil separating our existence from the place before and the place after. These moments of mystery challenge our understanding of "being." It is no coincidence that birth and death—the extremes of our existence—are the moments when we most honestly reconcile with ourselves.

I am fifteen weeks pregnant, with one daughter living, another daughter beyond this world, and a new baby brother for Havi and Kaia on the way. Soon we will be our own tragically beautiful family of five.

CHAPTER 53

Room 36

It is seven days before the one-year anniversary of that cold January morning when Havi took her last breaths in my arms.

We reserve the same room at the same inn on Cape Cod that we had with Havi this time last year. Room 36. We arrive on Friday morning, with Kaia. We walk across the lobby to the same elevator we rode up and down with Havi, and then down the same hallway to our room. The hotel smells of the ocean and fresh linen, same as last year. When I open the door to our room, I am flooded by emotions and memories. Tears fill my eyes as I bend down to grab our luggage from the cart. Once in the room, I look for Havi, seeing fleeting images of her everywhere: in front of the fireplace, where we put her rocker and watched her rest peacefully while we ate dinner, and over near the window where Matt danced with her to several tracks from an album by the band, Japanese Wallpaper. But most of all, I look for her on the bed, where Matt and I snuggled with her, the three of us wrapped in warm towels after a long shower together.

Now it's Saturday, 6:00 a.m., and still dark out. Today promises to be gray and rainy again. The porch is covered, but it's been raining all night and everything is wet. Kaia and Matt are the only ones out, waiting and watching for dawn to break. I can see she's asleep in the stroller and Matt is rocking it back and forth with his foot while sipping coffee on the patio. She had a rough night last night and ended up in our bed at 3:00 a.m., wide awake. So after early morning trade-offs between Matt and me, with both of us trying to get some sleep, Matt takes Kaia downstairs for a walk, gets a coffee from the lobby, tucks her into the stroller, and she is asleep in minutes. Just like Havi, Kaia sleeps really well when it's cold outside, and she likes being all bundled up inside the sleeping bag stroller liner.

Friday's raw weather persists so we stay inside as the day slides toward evening. We open the challah that we had picked up before we left and are happy to find that somehow a hint of the oven's warmth still clings to the soft loaf. We tear off pieces of the sweet bread and raise them in a toast: "To Hav. Always to Hav." Then we brace ourselves against the chill—even the ubiquitous seabirds look cold—and venture outside with Kaia over the snow-crusted sand to the same beach we strolled Havi before her death a year ago.

We etch Havi's name in the frozen sand like we do in every welcoming spot and hold each other for a few minutes. I peer into the stroller to make sure Kaia is okay. Matt turns to me, "Life with Havi physically here made the most sense of anytime in my life that I can remember. But at the same time, it made no sense at all. I feel like, when she was alive, she reached out her hand to me—*Dad, hold on here*—and pulled me through the fabric of space-time into another realm."

I say nothing. I look at Havi's name in the sand. Seeing and saying her name keeps her in the front row with us. And that's what we want: to allow Havi to exist in our ordinary day-to-day lives. So we watch until her name is slowly erased by the waves, knowing we'll write it over and over on every shore we visit.

> *"Memory is an invitation to the source of our life, to a*
> *fuller participation in the now."*
> DAVID WHYTE

My Hard-Learned Lessons about Grief

As you already know from reading my story, I have written to Havi every day since her diagnosis. I do this for myself. I have written this memoir for you. It is for you because implicit in our story are lessons in humanity that may benefit you. I have made them explicit and broadly applicable in this afterword; all of us have or will experience grief in our lifetimes. I hope my uninvited education provides guidance and succor when that inevitability arrives.

(1) Embrace Ritual

Rituals create intentional space for remembering and honoring loved ones who have died. They're organized ways to express our love and our pain, with our families, our community, or in private. Our capacity to cope grows when we let ourselves remember and feel in these sacred spaces. Rituals strengthen trust and connection with others, and with ourselves.

Rituals that honor major occasions in the wake of loss can buffer hurtful cues from the outside world that coax us to move on and "be happy." They can nourish our yearning for our beloved(s). These rituals aren't meant to distract or numb pain. Rather, they take us to the edge of our deepest pain, and our deepest beauty, so our hearts, our worldview, our community will deepen and expand.

Besides marking major occasions, ritual is also essential in our day-to-day lives. "Microrituals"[1] can happen as often or as infrequently as you need them. They recognize and promote *integration in grief.* Integrating the people who have died into our regular, everyday lives keeps us from *disintegrating.* When we disintegrate, we are literally "broken into parts;" we "lose our unity and integrity." These rituals are powerful in their simplicity:

---

[1] Joanne Cacciatore and Melissa Flint, "Mediating Grief: Postmortem Ritualization After Child Death," *Journal of Loss and Trauma*, 17:2 (2012), 158-172.

- *The presence of their absence:*[2] Say good morning to your loved one, out loud. Say goodnight to them, out loud.
- *Turn toward (rather than avoid)*: Choose one photograph each day, week, or month. Look at it closely; study the person's features. Trace your finger over their face. Close your eyes and *feel* them with you. Try to recall where you were when the photograph was taken. Let your mind and heart go to that time and place.
- *Music as a medium:* Listen to one song daily (or weekly) that reminds you of your person. Listen for how the lyrics move you. Let yourself be moved to tears if tears are what come. Don't judge yourself if they don't come today. Choose a new song every few weeks. Consider making a soundtrack of sacred songs that give you permission to feel.
- *Express yourself:* Write in a journal. Consider turning toward your loved one by addressing the entry to the person who has died. "Dear Beloved." Don't lift your pen from the paper—let your thoughts, feelings, and reflections come as they do. Tell your person what you did today.
- *Wear them:* If there is a particular color or pattern that evokes their presence, embrace it. Consider finding ways to always have a little bit of "purple" or "stripes" with you wherever you go.
- *Poetry as a medium:* Choose a weekly poem to meditate on; consider reading it out loud, as if you were speaking it to your beloved.
- *Include them:* Raise a glass to your beloved before dinner.
- *Indulge yourself:* Choose a special treat for one day of the week that has some connection to your beloved, i.e.: "Milkshake Mondays."

We can use ritual to embrace the symbolism of our grief. Symbols, colors, and meaningful physical manifestations of the people we've lost help us send our love for them out into the world. They serve as a reminder that our loved ones always exist.

---

[2] Joanne Cacciatore, *Bearing the Unbearable: Love, Loss, and the Heartbreaking Path of Grief* (Somerville, MA: Wisdom Publications, 2017). See, in particular, 115.

- *Embrace symbolism:* On a daily walk, notice nature's reminders of your people. They may "appear" to you as a heart-shaped leaf or in the beautiful shade of purple in the night sky. Trust how you feel in these moments. Whatever your belief system, embracing the mystery can be healing.

Names have real power, history, and meaning. Saying the names of the people we've lost integrates them into our everyday existence. Name them, speak of them, speak to them.

- For instance, you might order a coffee or tea or takeout in their name. Listen for how their name sounds when the barista calls it out, or how it looks on the bag when your food is delivered.
- Write their name in the sand, snow, dirt or clay. Use your finger or a stick. Do this in places you traveled together, and also in places they never had the chance to go. This brings them with you to new places, incorporating their presence into your current life. Sharing memories and stories about the people we've lost reinforces that their life mattered, and still matters, and makes their loss less ambiguous.

They EXIST.

Recall and share memories about the people we've lost from the physical world. Memories are our portal to their souls. Remembering helps keep them with us. Although it can be painful in the moment, it will ultimately soften the edges of our grief. Invite others to share memories, too. Sometimes other people's memories will spark new ones in you.

The word **remember** comes from re (again) – member (person within a community.) When we re-member, we maintain a connection to the person we've lost. When we do the opposite, we dis-member them. Dis (not, exclude, or cut-off) – member (person within a community). Fundamentally, remembering then, is about inclusion and connection; while dis-membering is about distancing ourselves or disconnecting. Disconnection is the root of loneliness. Acts of remembering are life sustaining for grieving people.

(2) It's Good to Feel

Honor your feelings: Honor whatever you are feeling right now: anguish, numbness, fear, despair, anger, impatience, withdrawal. Those emotions are organic. They emerge naturally. It is our loss, our tragedy, that is not normal. It is also okay to embrace the joy we may find in everyday moments or in ephemeral "encounters" with our dead.

Giving ourselves permission to feel is empowering. When we experience traumatic loss, we quickly learn that we control nothing. This realization can paralyze us with the sense of helplessness. Therefore, an essential practice in grief work is learning to let go, to accept our lack of control by accepting whatever we are feeling. To let our feelings be is to let them move through us. Movement is the opposite of paralysis.

Honoring our feelings is not easy. We are taught by our culture to run from pain, to move on from loss. We are told to be resilient, to get back to being the person we were before tragedy struck, to avoid talking about the person we've lost, to acquiesce to other people's comments about "silver linings" and "God's plans." We're encouraged to share only on other people's terms—giving others the power to dictate when and how we talk about the loss and pain that is ours, not theirs.

This narrative on grief is long overdue for a rewrite. Emotional repression keeps us from feeling—and that costs us our physical and mental well-being. Studies have found that "individuals who repress their emotions also suppress their body's immunity, making them more vulnerable to a variety of illnesses from common colds to cancer."[3] Like other stressors, repression affects immune function, the actions of the heart and vascular systems, and even the biochemical workings of the brain and nervous systems.

We can find relief in the theory of the "Unity of Opposites,"[4] which means holding two seemingly opposite feelings at the same time. Pain and pleasure coexist. Anguish and joy do not oppose, they amplify. Avoid either/or and instead, embrace a both/and worldview.

It's not sadness we should fear. What we should be afraid of is a "cult

---

[3] James W. Pennebaker, *Opening Up: The Healing Power of Expressing Emotions* (New York: The Guilford Press, 1997), 75-77, 139.

[4] Joanne Cacciatore, *Bearing the Unbearable*, 51-54.

of happiness"[5] that promotes superficiality over substance; parades perfection at the expense of meaning; and causes us to miss the opportunity to tap into a whole set of fiercely powerful emotions that could strengthen and enrich our connections to each other, and to ourselves.

When we embrace a constellation of feelings, we see awe and wonder alongside heartbreak; we better appreciate seemingly mundane moments. I am truly in awe of my two-and-a-half-year-old daughter who can put her own shoes on. I watch in sheer amazement as she finesses each of her shoes onto each of her feet. My older daughter did not live to do that. If I existed in an either/or world, watching my younger daughter put on her shoes would be painful alone, without the joy. And the reason I can experience awe is because I can experience anguish. While it might feel safe to avoid the depths of sorrow, doing so blocks our access to the epitome of pleasure. No one wants to exist in a gray and narrow place.

A second essential practice for honoring our feelings is to keep love close. There is no safe distance for loving. Keeping feelings at a distance can strain our bodies and close our hearts. Life is not eternal, but love is. When we love the one who's gone from us, they ARE.

Locked in silence, our grief will find a way to show up. Best to invite it in, embrace it, and then help it move with us.

(3) Movement Matters

The rhythmic tap of footfalls on the ground is a meditative practice that opens the mind, the heart and the soul, bringing us closer to what's real and raw in us. Movement through the natural world is transformative. It is freeing, liberating and empowering. There is no time when movement is needed more than when we are confronted with challenges in our life like grief and loss.

Moving is not a way to *move from* the hardest thing—like losing our first daughter—but a way to *move with* her.

Whatever your preferred form of movement is—walking, running, dancing, skipping, or jumping—some form of rhythmic, repetitive movement on a regular basis is essential to grief work. Dr. Bruce Perry's

---

[5] Joanne Cacciatore, *Bearing the Unbearable*, 25, 53, 80.

Neurosequential Model describes that "patterned, repetitive, rhythmic somatosensory experiences" regulate us so that we can access and connect to the parts of our brain that allow us to think and connect.[6]

Grief is physical. My arms literally ache from the absence of my daughter cradled in them. My legs are weighted by the fear that settles in them when I approach a playground filled with healthy children. And so, taking care of our bodies, being in touch with them, letting them move, and feeling where our points of tension are, enables us to notice what needs more attention.

Here's a series of "moving with" practices that can be easily integrated into ritualized walks or runs.

- *A silent or quiet mile*: If you are running or walking with a partner or a group of people, dedicate one mile (or any designated distance) to be in quiet. Use the time to remember, cry, laugh, or look for signs of your beloved. If you are by yourself, use this time to intentionally turn toward your beloved.
- *Take them with you:* Write their name on a piece of paper and put them in your sock, sports-bra, shorts pocket. Consider how it feels to "bring" them with you on this walk or run. What's different? What's the same? What does it bring up for you?
- *Look up and down:* Pay attention to where you are looking as you move. Have you ever looked all the way up to the tippy top of a tree? What comes up for you when you do? How much time do you spend looking at your feet? Are you present in your movement? Or are you always somewhere else?

These exercises might be challenging. If you've used movement as an escape or distraction, it can take time to integrate these practices. Also, *grief can get heavier before we learn how to move with it.* Be patient with yourself as you build your own emotional capacity to embrace and let it change you.

As we do hard things, we build mental and emotional muscle and stamina, and over time these "lifts" become lighter for us to carry.

---

[6] Bruce Perry and Eric Hambrick, "The Neurosequential Model of Therapeutics," *The Journal of Strengths-Based Interventions* (2008), 17.

Nature nourishes and regenerates: Nature is quiet, nonjudgmental and demands nothing from us, while inviting us to breathe and connect to a reality that is much bigger than ourselves.

Even looking up at the sky for a few minutes while swaying back and forth helps connect us to the big, mysterious world, grounding us in that bigger reality.

(4) Community Counts

While each person's grief journey is highly individual, connecting with people who make you feel good can be life-sustaining. Research shows that social support in grief helps with proactive coping and mitigates the intensity and duration of psychological distress and poor physiological outcomes. Education is power.

- While grieving people shouldn't have to be responsible for educating others, when we can muster up the energy to do so, it can serve us well. Read, study, examine grief as if it is your new best friend. Then, share the learnings that resonate with you—from your trusted scholars, grief counselors, poets, and spiritual leaders—with people with whom you'd like to be close. Send them books, poems, podcasts, or quotes.

Language liberates. Insist that people around you use language that integrates and honors your grief, rather than minimizing, colonizing, or avoiding it. For example:

- I am *with/loving/thinking of* you vs. I am *worried* about you.
- I know you will miss her *forever* vs. Time will heal.
- When I *try to imagine*, my chest tightens, and my throat starts to feel like it's going to close vs. I *can't* imagine
- It must be *impossible not to have your whole family* vs. *At least* you have *other* children.

Lastly, bear witness. When moments and memories are shared, witnesses are born. Invite others to become part of your sacred community: those who know the biography of your beloved. Include community members in rituals that become more powerful because they're shared.

Savvy Framework

You might want to use my "Savvy" framework for supporting a loved one who's grieving. The word savvy comes from the Latin verb *saber*: to know. Supporting someone in grief isn't about knowing, exactly; it's about feeling, intuiting. We can know and we can't ever know.

> **Savvy** = *Self-check, action-centered, vulnerable, values-based, year-round.*

- **S**elf-check: Consider who you are in relation to the person who is grieving. What is your role in their lives? What is your proximity to them and their beloved, emotionally and physically? What roles do you occupy in your own life that might make your support more or less helpful? Make sure your intentions are directed toward their needs; use language that draws them out and listen to what is being said, free of your own agenda.

- **a**ction-centered: Do things. Write things. Small things. Big things. All things. More is more. Of course, these need to be genuine acts of love and care with little self-focus. Send a text message with a photograph of a beautiful sunrise captioned, "thinking of you and your beloved." Send a hand-written note on a random day. Frame a photograph; share a memory; remember important dates; order food.

- **v**ulnerable: Derived from the Latin noun, *vulnus*, meaning "wound." Vulnerability begets vulnerability. People will only share and bear their souls to those of us who have earned their trust by demonstrating our own vulnerability. "I don't know how to be there for you, and it crushes me." "I feel lost in wanting to be better for you." "I am so afraid that I'm going to lose my daughter that I am afraid to be close to you." These are all invitations to the grieving person to share ways in which you might be able to be more helpful. The important thing is to make sure that they are framed in the context of wanting to be better for the GRIEVER. Be careful not to make this about YOU.

- **values:** Learn what matters to the person who you are supporting. What is most important to them in how they honor and integrate their beloved? What do they appreciate? What do they believe about faith or religion or spirituality? What do they not embrace? Align your support to THEIR values.

- **year-round:** The death of a child, and any significant loss, is not a one-time event, but one that happens every moment that the child, or person, is not where they are supposed to be. The losses are layered and continuous. They accrue every day, as well as on every missed milestone. You can send a "thinking of you" text message to the griever any time, any year, and it will be appreciated.

Savvy support is not a "crisis response" template. It is a way of being there for the people we love in a sustained way. It requires us to believe that staring straight at the most painful thing is the surest way to see with the greatest clarity and love.

ACKNOWLEDGMENTS

I owe an immense debt of gratitude to all the friends and family who supported us, and continue to do so, in holding Havi. Every act of kindness, courage, and generosity is deeply appreciated: every hand-written note, email, photograph, thoughtful wish, home-cooked meal, lantern lit, flower planted, t-shirt designed, circle held, donation made, mile run, muffin baked; every effort made to be with us for Havi's memorial service, and so many other acts of the most generous kind of humanity. I wish I could name them all, and you all. You keep us afloat.

Thank you to Lucia Knell for first sharing Havi's story with the world, for your beautiful and generous friendship, and for introducing me to my amazing agent, Emma Parry, who believed in an unknown author with no online platform, and who continued to advocate for this story despite persistent headwinds. And to Annalisa Quinn and Francis Storrs at the Boston Globe for believing in the power of Havi's story. Thank you to the Monkfish team: Paul, Jon, Colin, and Anne for ushering this book into the world with exquisite care and devotion.

Thank you to Meg Campbell who connected me to Beverly Donofrio and then to Susan Piperato. To Beverly for teaching me that "specificity is generosity," and firing me as her student so I would take the craft of writing more seriously. To Susan, our Wednesday afternoon meetings and every email exchange in between gave me the strength and conviction that I could write this book. I am forever grateful for your editorial talents, your friendship, your unwavering belief in the power of Havi's story, and your deep devotion to our family.

Thank you to Meredith Maran who, in the midst of making this a better book through her brilliance, experience, and wisdom, became a teacher, life-long friend, and trusted confidant. I know why she is considered the best in the business by Anne Lamott.

Thank you to Mary and Annie Connor for your friendship, encouragement, and contribution to early and ongoing phases of this book. You turned our CaringBridge entries into a real book and that inspired this memoir. I am forever grateful. And for the ways you show up as ever-present posse members in big and small ways all the time. And finally, for the gift of Havi's sacred bench that I wish I could have shared in this book.

Thank you to Lauren Markham for agreeing to read and endorse *Fifty-Seven Fridays* before I believed it could exist in the world. I have the deepest admiration for you as a human, mother, and writer and you should know that you catapulted this into the world. Thank you to Sarah Bailin for reading an early draft of this and sharing such thoughtful feedback. Thank you to Ellen Adams who I never had the chance to fully thank for her brilliant feedback on an early draft. And to Jackson Greenberg for making that beautiful connection. And to Marcy, Joel, Sara, Amnon, Alma, Josie, Ellie, and Henry for blessing us with your thoughtfulness and support from the time I was a little kid, through Havi's life and death, and every day since.

Thank you to Dr. Jo who is the source of so much of our wisdom. You are a gift to this world and teacher and guide for me. Thank you for embracing Havi's life alongside so many of the other beautiful children who you hold with such fierce compassion. And thank you to Michele Reimer for sharing *Bearing the Unbearable* with us. And for all the ways you cared for and care for my parents as they both ache and celebrate Havi.

Thank you to Greg Zaff for every walk and talk before, during and after Havi's death. You are a treasured mentor, friend, and confidant. Thank you to Rosemary McElroy for sharing so many gifts of wisdom and generosity with us—too many to name; for our refuge in NH, the Havi-Kaia Oak Tree, and your unwavering friendship. And for always knowing the right thing to say. And to the SQB family for honoring Havi's name so beautifully and thoughtfully; your devotion to Havi is extraordinary. Thank you to Barbara Weber for sharing the Tango family so generously with us and for every act of lovingkindness. And for Gigi de Manio, whose photographs line the walls of our home. Gigi, somehow the images capture even the softness of Havi's skin.

Thank you to Bonnie Hammer, god-mother extraordinaire. You were instrumental in helping me navigate this new world. Thank you to Michelle Notkin for every heart, challot, and purple outfit. And for our time with you in Ojai when Havi was swept up in your love. Thank you to Ossie for the countless acts of thoughtfulness—blueberry trays, knee pads, children books, and every note in between.

Thank you to Rob Levinthal for editing early sections that didn't make it into this book; I hope those pages find their way into another book. Our childhood, and our friendship, are foundational to the way I see the world. Thank you to Sam Charleston and Amanda Foote for every call, visit, and note that reassured me that Havi is forever. I wish you didn't have to know loss. To Kathleen and Heather for your unwavering devotion. To the Carstensens for all the ways you honor and integrate Havi. You are the most beautiful people.

Thank you to Rabbi Shelly for sharing sacred time, poetry, and prayer with me and Matt after Havi's death, and for continuing to find ways to bless her life through your beautiful Or Zarua congregation. Thank you to the E-motion community. Here's to as many sacred circles as we need.

To Uncle Dresh, for loving Havi whole-heartedly, and walking this with us. To Uncle Jesse for bringing a full spirit to every day at our home and for being the Uncle JJ that we, and our kids, need and love. And to Zoe and Nick, for every song, mile and red-tailed hawk sighting. You are forever posse-members. Thank you to Scotty, Carolyn, and the Young family: from the Swarthmore baseball field to Blaisdell Lake and back again. You have been a beautiful and constant presence for Matt and me. Your love is forever incorporated in the ink of Havi's heartbeat that lies on Matt's chest over his heart.

Thank you to Beverly Poling Cummins for holding Havi with such tenderness. We miss you. Bohmillers and Schneiders: For your biggest hearts. Eternal love, incredible cousins. Sack Aunts, Uncles, and Cousins. For your love and generosity always from near and far. And to Uncle Brodie who I wish could have held Havi; it would have been instant love.

Thank you to Allison Wolfe and the Wolfe family who keep Havi's essence alive through the most beautiful gifts of artwork, design, and drawings. Your challah cover and Lev blanket are ever-present in our home and literally wrap us in your love and thoughtfulness every week.

Thank you to Kelsey Quick (Aunt Kiki): There could have been chapters dedicated to all the big and small ways you were and are with us every day, carry Havi with you, enhance my life, and have become family. Thank you to Allison (Hubs) Hadley (Aunt Al), and Becky Poskin (Aunt B) who began as Dartmouth Soccer teammates and have become sisters and best friends. Thank you to Greg (Uncle Greg) and Lucas (Uncle Lucas) for appreciating the power and beauty in being married to DWSers. For the ways you each keep Havi infused in your lives through craft, movement, and every-day acts of kindness. You are all forever Havi's posse.

Thank you to Blyth, Charlie, Taylor, Cameron, Eliza, and Deirdre's family. You are perhaps the greatest source of light and love that we could have possibly imagined in our lives. Yours is a friendship that is beyond this world.

Thank you to Gricelda Diaz, our Tia, and your beautiful family: Fabian, Edward, Vicel, and Dani. You mean the world to us and you are forever a part of our family.

To my forever Grandmommy, Zadie, Grandma Yoo Hoo, and Grandpa Harold. You are with me always as the heartbeat of our family.

Thank you to Havi's cousins: Ayla for carrying your little cousin Havi so exquisitely. And to Havi's little cousins: Hannah, Sela, and Hali, I hope you each take strength in knowing that you have a big cousin who loves you beyond this world.

Thank you to our siblings and our parents: This book is you. I could never do justice to the fierce compassion, out-of-this world generosity, and every-day acts of heroism you showed and continue to show. Havi only knew love because of you. I will spend the rest of my life sharing my deepest gratitude. We love you beyond measure. You are my best friends and my family. How lucky?

And a special thank you to Kaia and Ezra: Though you can't know it now, you inspired me to write this book. Should you ever choose to read it, I hope we can talk all about it together. You are both loved beyond measure and you are the greatest gifts of my life.

Finally, thank you to Matthew Goldstein. There is no man like you. And I hope you know how proud and admiring I am of who you are, how you carry our beautiful children, and how you love and support me unconditionally. You are superman. Don't hide!

ABOUT THE AUTHOR

Myra Sack graduated with a B.A in government and All-American Honors in 2010 from Dartmouth College, where she captained the women's varsity soccer team. She earned a post-graduate Lombard Fellowship in Granada, Nicaragua with Soccer Without Borders. Following her lifelong passion for sports and social justice, Myra joined SquashBusters, Inc., in Boston in 2013, serving as their Chief Program and Strategy Officer. Myra has an MBA in Social Impact from Boston University and is trained as a Certified Compassionate Bereavement Care provider by Dr. Joanne Cacciatore. She serves on the Board of the Courageous Parents Network and is the Founder of E-Motion, Inc., a non-profit organization with a mission to ensure community is a right for all grieving people. A writer, coach, and activist, Myra and her husband Matt, live in Jamaica Plain, MA with their second daughter, Kaia, and son Ezra. Myra's oldest daughter, Havi, passed away on January 20, 2021 of Tay-Sachs disease.